DO YOU REALLY NEED EYEGLASSES?

Revised 1985 Edition

MARILYN B. ROSANES-BERRETT, PH.D.

CONTENTS

PREFACE   5

Better Sight Without Miracles   9

The Discoveries of a Doubting Doctor   18

How to Use Your Eyes   24

How to Benefit From Light   31

Relax with the Aid of Your Palms   38

Swing—and See Better   44

How to Correct Eye Defects   53

Can Crossed Eyes Be Straightened?   65

Additional Common Problems   72

Making Your Eyes See in 3-D   82

Recent Cases of Interest   98

The Wisdom of the East   106

How and Why the Eye Can See   114

The Eyes, the Body, and Psychotherapy   127

APPENDIX   133

WHAT THE TITLES MEAN

YOUR CHILDREN'S EYES

ACKNOWLEDGMENTS   140

PREFACE

As a physician, I have been closely associated with the sight-training methods described in this book, and I would therefore like briefly to discuss some important aspects of the method with the reader.

Life is often stressful, and stress is known to take a heavy physical and emotional toll. Stress is involved in such common ailments as duodenal ulcers, high blood pressure, allergies, and mental illness. Similarly, there is a very close relationship between our emotional state and the visual function. Indeed, when we consider the complexity of the work which the eyes must perform in modern life, it is remarkable how well the eyes adapt to new demands. Vision will tend to be relatively poor at the end of a tiring day, keener in the morning when we feel refreshed.

In the same way as exercises and relaxation techniques keep us physically fit, the techniques described in this book will tend to improve vision. Basically, the aim of

5

sight training is to help us to use our eyes in the most effective manner.

Physicians are primarily concerned with the diagnosis and treatment of established diseases of the eye. We pay far less attention to the equally important field of preventive medicine.

The techniques described in DO YOU REALLY NEED EYEGLASSES? will greatly help individuals with common refractory errors. Occasionally, even patients with severe eye diseases have derived considerable benefit from a combination of this method and ophthalmological care.

The patients described in this book have been carefully selected, and the techniques have been performed under close medical supervision. The relaxation techniques described are beneficial for most people. When done correctly, these techniques can only enhance vision. Patients who do not respond require re-evaluation from the organic and psychological point of view.

It is important to stress that this sight-training program must be approached with a positive attitude and motivation. Those individuals who have been most successful have approached the task with discipline and constant application. For the individual with a genuine desire to improve his vision, this book has much to offer.

VALENTINE W. ZETLIN, M.D.

Medical Director, Gestalt Center for Psychotherapy and Training

PREFACE TO THE REVISED EDITION

Since the first edition of this book was published, I have received many letters from people who have been able to improve their eyesight by using my approach to eye training. In this revised edition I would like to share with you new procedures and additional information on ways to improve your vision.

I have included a completely new chapter on eye exercises used in modern China that have had dramatic success there. We have adapted these techniques and used them successfully in our clinic in New York to help relieve a whole gamut of eye problems. I have also expanded the chapter on "The Eyes, The Body, and Psychotherapy" to explain more fully the relationship between vision and attitude, which is essential to greater sight improvement. Throughout, I have added or amended material to take into account new findings that we have incorporated into the eye training program at the clinic.

Finally, I have included new case studies of clients

who have been able, in recent years, to benefit from the program and this book. All this is to encourage you, the reader, to take the first step toward improving your own vision. Read with an open mind, commit yourself to a regular schedule of the program that fits your needs, and enjoy the world that begins to appear before your eyes.

Marilyn B. Rosanes-Berrett, Ph.D.

Founder and Executive Director, Gestalt Center for Psychotherapy and Training

BETTER SIGHT WITHOUT MIRACLES

You wear eyeglasses or, the chances are, you would not have picked up this book. You expect to wear them for the rest of your life, obtaining stronger lenses every couple of years, as your eyes grow weaker. But unless you are a rare case, you could learn to see better without glasses than you now see with them. So could most of the other 100 million Americans who wear glasses and the 8 million who use contact lenses, which are even more expensive. This book proposes to tell you how.

Before you dismiss the whole idea as just another wacky fad, consider the following case histories arising from my professional experience.

When I first met Mrs. H., she was 84 years old, virtually immobilized by obesity and arthritis, and blind. My compassion for her was surpassed only by my awe at the formidable challenge she presented. I could do nothing about her obesity or her arthritis, for I was not a physician;

but as an intern in the field of sight improvement, I was supposed to try to do something about her blindness. Mrs. H. was my first client outside the institute where I had been trained, and had I not known better, I might have suspected that she had been assigned to me to convince me that I had chosen the wrong profession.

Mrs. H.'s sight difficulties had begun ordinarily enough many years before with presbyopia, the so-called farsightedness that commonly afflicts the middle-aged. (Presbyopia is regarded as being due to a loss of flexibility in the muscles. The eye's structure is described on page 100.) Mrs. H.'s presbyopia had worsened with extraordinary rapidity and had been followed by the development of cataracts. In this disease—which gets its deceptively alluring name from an old belief that tiny waterfalls cascade down between the crystalline lens and the part of the eye called the iris—the lens becomes obscured in varying degrees. Mrs. H.'s crystalline lenses had become totally opaque, and in the standard treatment, had been surgically removed. The cataracts were then succeeded by three attacks of acute glaucoma, a disease in which fluids within the eye build up sometimes painful and often dangerous pressures on the eyeballs.

Mrs. H. had undergone five operations—three for glaucoma as well as two for cataracts—and the outcome had been total blindness. She could only distinguish between light and darkness. Glasses seemed out of the question—even the strongest lenses need something on which to work, and Mrs. H. appeared to have nothing.

I visited Mrs. H. once a week for 90 minutes in her flat just north of a New York district called Hell's Kitchen. She shared this apartment with an aged brother and an overworked widowed daughter who supported the family. On each visit, I instructed Mrs. H. in techniques designed to rejuvenate or improve sight, on the premise that she might yet have vestiges of vision of which she was unaware. Between my visits, Mrs. H. enthusiastically practiced—hour after hour—the procedures I had detailed. She had nothing else to do anyway, and she found these exercises to be pleasant pastimes.

Three months after my first visit, Mrs. H. could distinguish the table and chairs in her kitchen, and if the light was good, a vase and a bright-colored bowl. After six months of practice, she cried out gleefully one morning when she found she could read a headline in her brother's copy of the New York *Daily News*.

Within weeks, she was enjoying the color photographs in *Life* magazine and deciphering the largest captions.

Soon she began to play solitaire, then to write letters with big black crayons. Without glasses! Most important of all—at least to her daughter—she began to cook again, and though all of this took place almost 25 years ago, I can still savor the rice pudding she made for me as my reward. She was particularly proud of having been able to use the measuring cup correctly.

Five years later, when I had my last contact with her, she was able to read a newspaper for brief periods with

the help of strong lenses. And significantly, she was com-
plaining less about her arthritis, and she was moving
about much more than she did when I had first met her.

Mr. Q., a 65-year-old engineer who did most of his
work at a desk, was brought to me by his 75-year-old girl
friend, a nurse who was already my client. Mr. Q.'s ophthalmologist (see Appendix, page 114) had just informed
them that Mr. Q.'s glaucoma had reached a dangerous
level and required immediate surgery. They arrived at
the office understandably concerned, for the surgery
would permanently incapacitate Mr. Q. for his profession.
Could I do anything? With far more brashness than I
could muster today, I said: "I'll try—if you can give me
eight hours a day for two weeks."

For the next fortnight, eight hours a day, Mr. Q. followed procedures somewhat similar to those Mrs. H. had
practiced. On the fifteenth day, Mr. Q. returned to his
ophthalmologist. The glaucoma had subsided. The operation was postponed indefinitely.

And Mr. Q. found he could now see well with an old
pair of glasses much weaker than those he had been using.
He continued to apply the techniques he had learned
during those two weeks; and in the eight years up to his
death of a heart ailment, he had not suffered a recurrence
of glaucoma.

Mrs. L. was 41, and on the recommendation of several ophthalmologists, was preparing to study Braille in

expectation of total blindness. For ten years she had suffered acute attacks of choroiditis, an inflammation of a middle lining of the eyeball. Her doctors had administered both orthodox and experimental treatments, including doses of cortisone and of various antibiotics, but the left eye was already sightless, and the right eye was failing.

Mrs. L. came to me skeptically, and only at the insistance of her husband and her sister. I gave her two lessons, and I released her on her promise to practice for the next three months what she had been taught. At the end of three months, she wrote to me. Her ophthalmologist had told her that her chroiditis had been arrested and that the damaged tissue seemed to be healing. With weak glasses, she could see better than she had seen with stronger glasses prescribed for her even before the onset of choroiditis.

When Mrs. L. told her doctor what she had been doing, he sniffed: "Christian Science"—which with all due respect for Christian Science, it was not. Now in her sixties, Mrs. L. holds a responsibile corporate post that requires much careful reading. She still practices the techniques she learned in her first two lessons, often without even thinking about them, and her choroiditis was arrested.

Mrs. Z. was in her late fifties or early sixties, I judged, when she traveled from Atlantic City to Florida, where I was then teaching. Her doctor had informed her that she was beginning to develop cataracts. Just to make sure, she had consulted a second ophthalmologist, who had confirmed the diagnosis.

I gave her two lessons, four days apart, before she left on a six-week cruise. During the voyage, she practiced assiduously the techniques I had taught her. On her return, she visited the doctor who had first noted the incipient cataracts. He examined her and said: "I must have diagnosed you incorrectly. I don't see any sign of cataracts now."

She replied: "No, you were right, doctor. After you saw me, I consulted another eye doctor and he confirmed your diagnosis."

The doctor shook his head. "It never happens," he said. "Cataracts don't disappear."

Mrs. Z. then began to tell him of the techniques she had used aboard ship. Less polite than Mrs. L.'s doctor, who had dismissed Mrs. L.'s experience as "Christian Science," Mrs. Z.'s doctor cut her short with "Poppycock!"

Poppycock or not, 10 years later Mrs. Z. was still daily employing the techniques of sight training, and when I last heard from her she had not developed cataracts. Neither did she suffer from presbyopia, which had also afflicted her when we first met.

The case of Mr. C., who is well known in broadcasting, is less dramatic than those I have recounted, but it is the only case I know of that involved training by telephone. Mr. C. was about 25 when I first saw him. His case was not much of a challenge, because he had only moderate myopia, but he endeared himself to me by working so hard between his weekly visits that he showed an improvement in vision each time he came to me. After 20 lessons, he needed no more training—his myopia was gone.

Although Mr. C. referred a couple of clients to me, I did not hear from him directly for several years. Then he telephoned me, long distance. His young child had a marked cast in one eye, he said, and surgery was being considered to correct it. What did I think? Over the phone, I described techniques that I had found useful in such cases. A series of long distance telephone conversations followed in the next few weeks. I never saw the child; but after several months, Mr. C. reported that the child's condition had improved greatly.

And then there was my own case. At 27, I suffered from three defects of vision. I had hyperopia—known also as hypermetropia—in which rays of light entering the eye converge behind the retina rather than on it. Victims of hyperopia are often described as farsighted because they see distant objects better than those close up; but in fact, their distant vision is seldom better than average. I suffered, too, from astigmatism. This is another very troublesome error of refraction. In this condition, instead of the cornea being spherical, it is a little flatter than usual. This flatness is perhaps due to pressure of the lids on the globe, or tensed muscles. And to complicate my plight, I had a mild case of strabismus—crossed eyes or squint. When I was tired, my right eye manifested a cast, and my vision failed to merge into a single picture of what each eye saw separately.

I felt oppressed by unrelenting eyestrain. My doctors prescribed even stronger glasses, and my sight worsened steadily. My morale had ebbed to a lifetime low when a friend, Sidney Fields, a newspaper columnist, told me there was a way to improve my sight that did not depend on glasses: his young son was getting such training. On his recommendation, I sought out an organization then known as the American Association for Eye Training. Almost incredibly, after a single lesson I saw better and my sense of strain vanished. After several lessons, I discarded my glasses.

Today, more than 23 years later, I still do not need glasses, although most people my age have long since resorted to wearing them.

My experience as a client led me to study sight training, and to qualify to pass on the techhniques that had helped me and many (though by no means all) of the people who had applied these techniques. Those techniques appear so simple that a friend of mine jestingly compares them to kicking a non-working radio and hearing it burst into Mahler's Second Symphony. One technique that helped Mrs. H., for example, merely required her to sit in front of an ordinary incandescent lighted lamp, shut her eyes gently, and turn her head slowly from side to side. In another procedure, she had only to cover her eyes with her palms for 20 minutes at a time.

Among the techniques I devised for Mr. Q., the one most likely to elicit the comment "Aw, come on, now!" consisted of having his nurse wave a colorful magazine before his eyes several times a day. (In glaucoma, from which Mr. Q. suffered, the functioning area of the eye may become constricted. When Mr. Q.'s eyes followed the movement of the magazine, they broadened the functioning area, bit by bit, until that area extended to the entire periphery.)

These techniques are described in detail in later chapters, with instructions for applying them and with explanations of why they often succeed.

THE
DISCOVERIES
OF A
DOUBTING
DOCTOR

The techniques of sight training evolved from the discoveries, as far back as 75 years ago, of Dr. William H. Bates, a distinguished New York ophthalmologist who became one of the most controversial figures in modern medicine. Bates seemed an unlikely wave-maker. A graduate of Cornell and of the College of Physicians and Surgeons in New York, he instructed doctors in ophthamology at the New York Post-Graduate Medical School and Hospital. He frequently was summoned as a consultant on baffling eye problems. His hospital connections were impressive, including at various times Bellevue, Harlem Hospital, Manhattan Eye and Ear Hospital, and New York Eye Infirmary. He practiced his profession for years with impeccable orthodoxy.

But in the course of examining some 30,000 pairs of eyes a year, Bates became increasingly disturbed over the fact that what he observed often contradicted what he had been taught, and what he was teaching. One major anomaly involved the eye's ability to shift focus from distant to nearby targets and vice versa, a process that optical science calls accommodation. Poor accommodation equals poor vision—manifesting itself in nearsightedness, farsightedness, presbyopia, and other malfunctions.

Ophthalmologists were sure they knew how accommodation worked. Ever since 1851, when the German scientist, physiologist, and philosopher Hermann Ludwig Ferdinand von Helmholtz invented the ophthalmoscope and used it to peer into the living eye, the explanation had been dogma: the crystalline lens provided accommodation by changing its shape, probably—though not even von Helmholtz was certain of this—in response to movements of the ciliary muscle. The job of the crystalline lens is to bend—technically, to refract—rays of light on their way to the retina. If refraction proves faulty, producing a vision malfunction, then—the reasoning went—the lens may be too thick, or too thin, or too hardened by aging to function properly. If nothing can be found wrong with the lens, then the ciliary muscles may be weak. In either case, prescribe glasses.

But, Bates asked, if it is the lens that provides accommodation, why do eyes accommodate properly after the lens has been removed, as it is in an operation for cataract?

Bates also questioned the accepted view that the shape of the eyeball, once fixed, never changes. When the eyeball is too short from front to back it produces hyperopia—farsightedness, or longsightedness, as Britons call it. When the eyeball is too long, the result is myopia—

nearsightedness, or shortsightedness. In either case, the eye behaves like a badly focused camera, and by the rule book of ophthalmology, nothing can be done about it except to prescribe glasses. But, said Bates, I have seen hyperopia and myopia come and go, and my patients are able to see better on some occasions than on others. The eyeball, he argued, must be able to change its shape.

Bates plunged into research that lasted 40 years. Among the conclusions he reached are:

Defective vision and even such diseases as glaucoma may be influenced by emotional stress and strain. Our eyes do not fail us, we fail them. Relaxed and healthy, we see at our best, which is not necessarily so good as somebody else's best. Tense, tired or ill, we see at our worst. (Where tension or trauma reach extremes, as in miliary combat, total blindness may develop in people with normal eyes.)

Avoid strain, relieve stress—and sight will improve, sometimes with astonishing rapidity, sometimes slowly. Strain can be avoided by the adoption of certain simple habits in using the eyes. Stress can be relieved by practicing relaxation techniques.

Though growing older is inevitable, presbyopia—the farsightedness that most people develop in their forties—is not. With aging, we lost flexibility of the muscles, and the eyes are thus less able to accommodate and converge.

Myopia and hyperopia—nearsightedness and farsightedness—are not permanent, irremediable disabilities determined by the fixed shape of the eyeballs. Their shape is not fixed—it can change constantly in response to many factors, among them tense muscles. If an eyeball does not change its shape, it is because those muscles are tense from strain, and hold it rigid, or are flaccid from disuse or misuse, and exert no effort.

Eyeglasses generally do more harm than good. They are intended to correct errors of refraction—the bending of light rays to focus the rays on the retina. But instead, glasses perpetuate those errors. Errors are inherent in the eye; the eye makes them all the time, especially when looking at unfamiliar objects, but usually corrects them instantaneously. Glasses may make reading more comfortable, but they act as a "crutch," and do not treat the underlying cause of the visual error.

Bates opposed the use of eyeglasses with such conviction that he snatched them away from new patients and smashed them. In 1912, he vigorously fought a proposal to fit large numbers of New York City school children with glasses. As a result of his unorthodoxies, the American Medical Association dropped him from membership without announcing why. (Privately, the association charged him with "unethical advertising," but cynics cited pressure from the multimillion-dollar optical industry as the real reason for Bates's ouster.)

Although Bates, in effect, challenged the AMA to investigate his theories and prove him wrong, the AMA never did. Bates died in 1931, his theories neither disproven nor accepted by his colleagues. Anyone given to believing that most evils are rooted in vast conspiracies might easily blame the AMA's ostracism of Bates on the optical industry—which, indeed, years after Bates's death, was revealed to be paying generous kickbacks to professional men who prescribed glasses. But there are other rational explanations for Bates's differences with his colleagues.

Medicine is, and must be, a conservative profession, wary of new ideas until they have proven themselves. Sometimes, as in the case of Louis Pasteur, this caution can prove excessive. From a practical point of view, it is far easier for a busy doctor to prescribe eyeglasses than to undertake sight training which may require many months. After all, glasses have been helping man to see for a long time. The Chaldeans of the Bible are supposed to have employed some kind of lens for magnification. Nero watched gladiators battle through a gem he used as a kind of lorgnette. The Chinese of the 10th century read with the use of glasses. Roger Bacon wrote about eyeglasses in 1268, about the time that the Florentine Salvino degli Armati was supposed to have introduced them in Europe. Why abandon a time-tested, efficient device in favor of a new theory? Anyone whose glasses fog in the kitchen or whose work day is ruined because of glasses forgotten at home might answer the question differently. So might the millions who need ever stronger prescriptions because glasses weaken rather than strengthen their eyes.

Those, however, are not the reasons orthodox ophthalmologists cite when they scoff at Bates. They point, understandably, not to the successes of the Bates method

—like those with Mrs. H., Mr. Q., and Mrs. L.—but to its failures.

Bates was a magnificent pioneer; but like most pioneers, he merely opened up the territory. He could not explore it fully. Since his death, many new techniques have been devised to supplement those that he prescribed for relaxing the mind and body, and some of these new techniques are incorporated in this book. But more importantly, some tensions are so deeply ingrained within us that simple relaxing techniques fail to reach them. In such cases, a different kind of therapy is essential, and that kind of therapy, too, is discussed later in this book. In any case, improved sight is within the reach of millions of people—without glasses.

HOW
TO USE
YOUR
EYES

Even the healthiest and most relaxed of us do not enjoy perfect sight all the time. Nobody does. The eyes function faultlessly only when they are completely at rest, and never for longer than a few consecutive minutes, even while we sleep. But when you reach the end of this paragraph, you can take a long stride toward achieving better sight more of the time. At that point—the end of the paragraph—put down this book for a moment. If you are wearing glasses, take them off—but despite Dr. Bates's example, do not toss them away just yet. Look out the window. Let your eyes rove as far as they can, whether it is only to an apartment house a couple of blocks away or across fields to the horizon. Do not try to encompass the whole panorama at once in a stare; look at one point momentarily, glide to another and another, like an Indian scanning a plain for antelope. Try to see a small area clearly, while maintaining awareness of the whole field. Do *not* strain to see. Relaxation is essential to good vision, and the more you strain, the less you will see. If you cannot clearly see what you are looking at, shut your eyes for a few seconds, relax, and breathe deeply. (The eyes need oxygen and falter without it.) When you open your eyes, your vision will be sharper. Now bring your vision back into the room, to glance at a corner of the ceiling, at a picture on the wall, at an ashtray on the coffee table. The frequent and easy changes of focus will loosen the eye muscles. When you resume reading—you may put on your glasses again—let your eyes glide lightly over the type, without strain. Do not drive yourself to read rapidly. Keep the pace leisurely—you will enjoy more whatever you are reading, comprehend it better, and avoid fatigue. Look up from the page every so often to look out the window again and to glance around the room. Let yourself blink—not by doggedly clamping together the eyelids, but by letting them close gently and naturally. Blinking bathes the eyes in a soothing but potent antiseptic fluid compared with which the eyewashes sold in drugstores are, well, just so much eyewash. But don't think about blinking—it should just happen. Shut your eyes for a few seconds whenever you turn a page. The eyes thrive on work if they get frequent rests.

Reading by day, sit close to a window in a position that lets light fall unobstructed on your book. Do not worry that on a gray, wintry afternoon the light may be insufficient: if you can read comfortably, there is enough light. (The more relaxed you become—as you should if you follow the suggestions in this chapter—the less light you will need.) By night, avoid reading in a darkened room beneath a circle of light from a single lamp—no matter that our forefathers had to and survived. Keep the rest of the room softly lit, and stand your reading lamp to your left and slightly to your rear. When you look up from your page to glance around the room, the variation in the intensity of light will benefit your eyes. Some people find this troublesome at first; but in the long run, the results are worth any temporary discomfort.

The best place to read is wherever you are most at ease. Forget what your mother told you about sitting erect in a straight-backed chair. You can read just as well, or better, lying on a couch or propped against a pillow in bed, as long as you can breathe freely and have enough light. Forget, too, the injunction about keeping the page precisely in front of you, 14 inches from your nose. Hold the book wherever you see it best—to the right or the left if you wish—but shift it from time to time for change of focus.

Avoid reading when you are tired or ill. If you must read then, do it only for brief periods punctuated by frequent rests.

When you forgo reading to watch television, do not turn off all the lights: keep the room softly illuminated. And do not stare fixedly at the screen—keep your eyes gliding from one point on the screen to another and another. The eyes normally shift 80 times a second, and staring impedes their movement dangerously. Look away from the screen momentarily to glance around the room, for change of focus. Shut your eyes occasionally—you probably will not miss much—and blink frequently. Viewed that way, television—no matter what it may do to your mind—will not hurt your eyes.

Follow the same procedures at the movies—glide your eyes about the screen instead of trying to encompass the whole image at once. (You may notice that you see best one area and the field immediately surrounding it.) If you go to the movies often, sit farther back or farther forward—depending upon whether you are nearsighted or farsighted—than you did the last time.

In sight training, I have used movies as part of the course, seating nearsighted clients—with their glasses off —in the fifth row the first night, in the sixth row the second night, and progressing backward until they could see well from far in the rear. For the farsighted, the nightly shift was screenward. Occasionally, change your focus: if you're nearsighted, shift your gaze from the screen to the row of heads in front of you; if you're far-sighted, look up at the ceiling.

In other activities where you have previously worn glasses, take them off from time to time and go without them as long as you can do so comfortably. Since the quality of vision can change with astonishing rapidity, you may have flashes in which you see perfectly without glasses. Such flashes can be great morale boosters for people who fear they will never see well.

When you go walking, look at the world as though it were a television screen or a movie. Keep your eyes gliding, to a point in the distance, to a bird in a nearby tree, to the face of a pretty girl, or to a handsome man passing you, to a cloud. Never wear dark glasses, no matter how bright the day, unless a doctor has prescribed them as essential in treating an ailment. Though doctors often write prescriptions for dark glasses merely because patients request them, prolonged darkness is as bad for the eyes as light is good for them. Dark glasses induce an abnormal sensitivity to light, and eventually make light intolerable. Sailors who work on deck and scan the sea all day never wear dark glasses and yet retain good sight into old age, but their fellows in the engine room, toiling in dim light, frequently develop cataracts and other serious disorders of the eyes. The donkeys that were used to haul coal in the mines went blind in the dark, but regained their sight when they were retired to pasture. So don't be a donkey in a coal mine if you don't have to be. No dark glasses.

When you drive an automobile, do not "glue your eyes to the road." Look off to the horizon momentarily but frequently, then back to the highway just ahead, to the gauges on the dashboard, and then to the road again. Swivel your gaze from one side of the road to the other; simultaneously, keep aware of the fields of vision surrounding the focal points, although you will see those fields less clearly. Driving at night, do not look directly at the headlights of approaching cars—keep your eyes moving and evade the glare by glancing to the sides of the lights or below them.

If you ride buses or trains where seats face sideways rather than forward, as in New York, do not stare at someone across the aisle even if your stare is blank. Keep the eyes moving; it is not only better manners but better visual practice.

There is nothing mysterious about using our eyes in such ways. The facts have been available for many years, yet they are depressingly little known. For example, I showed a rough draft of this chapter to a writer friend who has lived a long time and read and traveled widely, but had never heard of good visual techniques. He tried to conceal his skepticism, but failed. When I met him again a few days later, he confessed: "I did not take what you wrote very seriously, but I tried your advice out of curiosity. I was working at home and I began to look up from my typewriter to gaze out the window and to cast my eyes around the room. And I closed my eyes a lot. When I quit work at the end of the day, I cleaned up my desk and came across a note I had forgotten about. I read it through, and when I put it down I must say I was surprised to find that I was not wearing my glasses. First time in 30 years that I have been able to read anything smaller than a newspaper headline without glasses."

He will do even better if he makes good visual techniques a habit—so much of a habit that he practices them without thinking about them, as does Mrs. L., our friend from Chapter 1, who still sees well in her sixties. If every child in the country were instructed in those techniques early, if every adult could be convinced of their value, we might soon cease to be a nation in which glasses are worn by almost 10 percent of people under 16, almost 32 percent of those between 17 and 44, and almost 59 percent of those over 45. These figures are the worst in the world —and the answer is not that Americans get better eye care than other people do. We do not. We simply depend more on glasses; and in so doing we destroy our vision.

HOW TO
BENEFIT
FROM
LIGHT

Good visual habits are a first step, but only a first step, toward better sight. The steps that follow on the path consist of the practice of techniques that relax the mind and body, improve blood circulation to the eyes and brain, loosen tensed muscles—including those of the eyes —and tauten flaccid muscles.

These techniques—which emphatically are *not* exercises—have been found to banish or alleviate nearsightedness, farsightedness, presbyopia, and other common malfunctions. When they fail, it is because they have been faultily executed, or because the visual defects are deeply rooted in the mind—for the eye is an extension of the brain—and psychotherapy may be called for.

A few of these techniques were devised by Dr. Bates, and some by teachers who followed him; but many in this book represent new procedures, or deviations from old ones, developed of necessity in the course of my work.

SUNNING

Among the most fundamental and most generally useful of these techniques is one called Sunning, which consists simply of bathing the eyes in light—natural or artificial. It is based on the interrelated facts that (1) the eyes flourish on light and (2) they see by the contrast between light and darkness: the more light the eyes are exposed to and learn to accept, the more efficiently they function in good light or bad. Sunning provides light. But its effects are astonishingly broad.

Sunning is, first, a relaxant for mind and body, so it benefits everyone, keen eyes or dull.

For people afflicted with myopia, hyperopia, presbyopia, Sunning loosens the tightened muscles responsible for these malfunctions. For those suffering from strabismus, Sunning has uncrossed eyes at least temporarily, and sometimes to a great degree.

Sunning stimulates the retina, which grows dim and insensitive if it is long deprived of light. Light is food for the retina and other nerve tissue essential to sight. Deprived of light, the retina starves—which is one powerful reason I so strongly oppose dark glasses and favor Sunning. (Sunning rejuvenated parts of Mrs. H.'s scarred and atrophied retina; and to a considerable extent, accounted for her recovery of some sight.)

There is a theory that Sunning, because it stimulates the retina, slows the aging of the brain. The theory is based on the fact that (1) when stimulated, the retina transmits images to the brain along one large nerve, and then along several other nerve pathways to the visual site at the back of the brain; (2) these nerves are essentially parts of the brain; (3) when in use, these nerves set up reverberations in other brain nerves in related areas; (4) active nerves mean an active brain. Active brains, like active muscles, last longer.

Sunning banishes photophobia, the sensitivity to light that impels many people to wear dark glasses that make them still more photophobic.

And less dramatically, Sunning clear bloodshot eyes, helps overcome and prevent granulation of the eyelids, and eliminates itching of the eyes. (Never rub itching eyes —Sun them instead.)

Yet for all its good works, Sunning is the most undemanding of practices. Sunning is as pleasant and soothing as a warm bath for the body. Sunning in sunlight is more effective in the long run than Sunning by artificial light, but the eyes must become accustomed to Sunning slowly and gradually. So in your first few weeks of Sunning, better stick to the manufactured variety of light.

To practice Sunning, you will need only a comfortable, straight-backed chair; an ordinary, incandescent pole lamp—never, *never* use a sun lamp, a heat lamp, or a fluorescent light for Sunning—and an incandescent light bulb.

Begin with a wattage that is comfortable for your eyes (usually a 25- or 40-watt bulb is best) in a lamp placed between three and six feet away from you. If you are past your middle years, it is very important to protect your eyes by starting with no more than 25-watts at six feet. Gradually, week by week, increase the wattage from 25- to 40-, 60-, 100- and finally 150-watt bulbs. When you reach 150-watts you may want to try using a reflector spotlight for a greater concentration of light. Remember, increase the wattage only as your eyes become accustomed to the stronger light. To put your equipment to work and begin Sunning, see Figure 1 and follow these steps:

(1)   Set the lamp three to six feet in front of your straight-backed chair, screw the bulb into the socket, and switch on the light.

(2)   Seat yourself comfortably in the straight-backed chair with your back erect, your feet flat on the floor, and your nose pointed straight ahead, not up or down.

(3)   Take off your glasses and close your eyes gently. (No squeezed-down eyelids, please.)

(4)   Now turn your head slowly, smoothly, and rhythmically from side to side, midway to each shoulder, but no farther—too long a turn will tense the neck muscles and one of the objectives of Sunning is to relax your muscles.

(5)   Let the light soak into your closed eyes as your turning head passes through the glow. Feel your

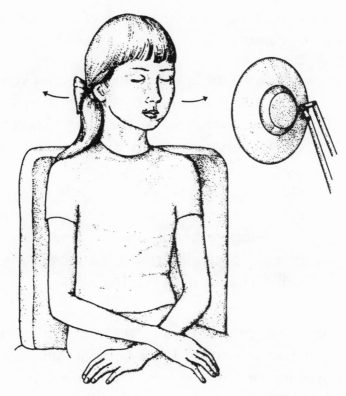

Figure 1.

In Sunning, the lamp should be centered directly in front of the face. In this Figure, the lamp has been drawn on the side so as not to obscure the face.

whole head move slowly and loosely, like the pendulum of a stately grandfather clock. Become aware of the many tiny muscles that join the back of your head to your neck; help them relax by imagining that you are breathing into them. Focus also on the muscles in front of your

ears, that control your jaw. Loosen them by
yawning.

(6)   Restrict your first few Sunnings to five minutes.
Over the period of a month, work up to twenty
minutes a sitting, if you can. This gives your
whole nervous system time to relax, too. Sunning seems to work much more effectively for
older people when it is done in a few twenty-
minutes sessions, rather than many brief periods. Younger people, on the other hand, appear
to benefit equally from a few long or many short
daily sessions with the light.

Once you are thoroughly at ease with the reflector
spotlight, you are ready for a bath of sunlight—out-of-
doors, by an open window, or even through a window-
pane. Restrict a natural sunbath to four minutes at a
time. Keep your nose level; don't raise your eyes to the
sun. And despite the counsel of Dr. Bates and some
other teachers, do not blink at the sun or open your eyes
and look at it. Without expert guidance, such practices
promote staring and prolonged focusing, both detrimen-
tal to the eyes.

When performed in the manner described in these
pages, however, Sunning is perfectly safe and usually en-
genders a sense of well-being. Occasionally, novices at
Sunning will experience nausea or uneasiness. If that happens to you, do not give up quickly: the discomfort gener-

ally passes. But if it persists, Sunning is not for you and psychotherapy may be necessary.

Because light is good for the eyes, avail yourself of it even when you cannot perform the Sunning procedure. Walk on the sunny side of the street and don't worry about glare: if the light is so strong that you find yourself tightening your forehead and tensing your eyelids, gently close your eyes part way. When you have become a veteran at Sunning, glare probably won't bother you any more than it bothers a seaman—and you will not only see better but also feel better all over.

RELAX WITH
THE AID OF
YOUR
PALMS

After Sunning, Palm. Even if you have not tried Sunning, Palm.

Palming consists of cupping the hands gently over the eyes, a technique which, like Sunning, is not an exercise in the sense of strained activity. Palming epitomizes inactivity: its purpose is to relax mind and body thoroughly and to rest and revitalize the eyes. Palming is particularly important after Sunning because it improves circulation to the eyes and surrounding structures. Adequate circulation is essential for normal visual function. Good circulation is particularly important when we reach middle age and beyond.

You can Palm almost anywhere—at home in a chair or in bed, in your office at a desk, in an automobile, on a train, or on an airplane. But to benefit you, Palming must be performed in a prescribed manner.

Palming at home, you will need only a pillow. Traveling, you may substitute a briefcase or a small suitcase. In your office, your desk should suffice. To Palm, see Figure 2 and follow these steps:

(1)   Start with warm hands. Cold hands will repel the flow of blood to the eyes, warm hands will accelerate that. If your hands are cold, warm them by rubbing them together, or by shaking them vigorously.

(2)   Sit erect in a comfortable but straight-backed chair.

(3)   Place a pillow or its substitute on your lap, and rest your elbows on it to support your upper arms. If you are lying in a bed or on a couch, rest your head on one pillow and put another across your chest for your arms.

(4)   Close your eyes gently.

(5)   Relax your hands, and cup your palms lightly over your eyes, with the sides of your hands against the sides of your nose, and the overlapping fingers on your forehead. Although there should be no pressure on the eyeballs, no light should reach your eyes if you Palm correctly.

(6)   As you Palm, let your mind drift to a pleasant memory—a day of peaceful fishing in a forest lake, a night stroll among the illumined foun-

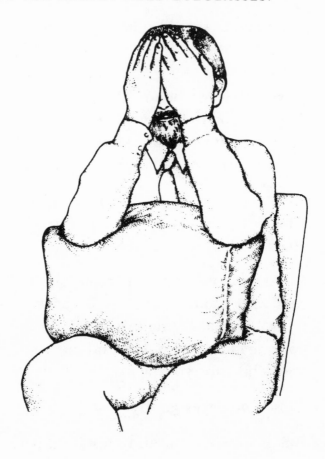

Figure 2.

tains of Rome's Tivoli, a high school picnic, or
any other cherished recollection.

(7)   Don't strive to recall details—let your mind vol-
unteer them. Palming is a form of constructive
meditation, and effort—even the effort to remember—will negate the relaxation which is a

purpose of Palming. For this reason, I disagree with Dr. Bate's recommendation that while Palming you should try to "see black." If you do see black, good—you have reached the pinnacle in Palming. But don't consciously work for it. At the start, you will probably see gray rather than black.

(8) If you feel restless while Palming, stand up and shake yourself gently—the restlessness should disappear. If your arms get tired, lower them, shake them, or move them rhythmically. Then resume Palming.

When the eyes feel tired or particularly heavy, combine Sunning and Palming. Palm to a slow count of 10. Then Sun to an equally slow count of 10. Repeat the Palming and Sunning alternately for four more counts each, slowly, without tension. Your eyes will see better and you will feel better.

Palm as often as you can, as long as you can. Even five minutes of Palming during a busy day at the office will refresh you and your eyes. Whether you find time to Palm at the office or not, be sure to Palm for at least 20 minutes in the evenings. Palm when you have a headache—it will ease the pain. If you have serious eye defects, Palming more than 20 minutes a day would be beneficial.

Dr. Bates recounts a tale of a patient who undoubtedly established and must still hold a world record for unbroken Palming. The man, who was then close to 70, suffered from hyperopia—astigmatism and presbyopia—and was developing cataracts. He had worn glasses for 40 years, but had reached the point where he no longer could see well enough to work. Bates prescribed Palming, and the patient asked: "Can I do it too much?" Bates said: "No, Palming is simply a means of resting your eyes."

The patient returned a few days later, and said, "Doctor, it was tedious, very tedious, but I did it." He had Palmed continuously for 20 hours, pausing only to drink water but not to eat.

When Dr. Bates tested his eyes without glasses, the patient read the bottom line of the standard eye-test chart at 20 feet, and read small type at six inches and at 20 inches. Examination disclosed that the beclouding of the man's crystalline lenses—the manifestation of cataract—had lessened considerably. Two years later, the opacity had not deteriorated.

A final word about Palming. Not everyone finds it easy to relax while Palming. Most of us fill our minds most of the time with worries, plans, and thoughts of things we *should* be doing. If you have trouble freeing your mind from such thoughts, try focusing on yourself in a new way for a moment. Become aware of your breathing. Don't try to change it, just observe your breath coming in and going out of your body. Generally your breathing will become calmer of its own accord as you do this. Then you will begin to feel more relaxed and able to let pleasant memories come up. If you still feel restless, I suggest that you use something other than Palming right now and read the chapter "The Eyes, The Body, and Psychotherapy" for further suggestions on relaxation.

SWING—
AND SEE
BETTER

In his classic *Dance of Life*, Havelock Ellis wrote of the "rhythm which marks, not only life, but the universe." The surf beats rhythmically against the shore. Trees sway rhythmically in the wind. There is rhythm in the flight of a bird, the hum of a mosquito, the swing of elephants' trunks, the traffic patterns of the stars and planets. Men living close to nature—African tribesmen, American Indians, South Sea islanders—worship their gods with the rhythm of their dances. In the days of sailing ships, seamen would raise giant sails to the rhythm of the chantey.

But modern men and women in a technological age have lost touch with these primal rhythms; we are forever out of step inwardly and outwardly: we do not march, we straggle and stumble, figuratively. Swinging movements of the body revive physical and mental rhythms, engender harmony with the world—and thus enable us to see better.

Among the best of such swinging movements is the

Long Standing Swing. It is a relaxant: performed at bed-time, the Long Standing Swing makes for a restful night and has been known to banish insomnia. It stimulates blood circulation. Performed in the morning on rising, it makes the challenges of the work day ahead seem far less forbidding. If the Long Standing Swing can be crowded in during the day—ideally after you have Sunned and Palmed—it makes for a refreshing rather than a fatiguing afternoon.

Apart from its general tonic effect, the Long Standing Swing benefits the eyes, especially in myopia, presbyopia, and strabismus (commonly called squint or crossed eyes). Dr. Bates, who devised the Long Standing Swing as well as Sunning and Palming, reported that the Swing resulted in some improvement in sight even in cases of diplopia—double vision—and polyopia, or multiple vision.

For your first few experiences of the Long Standing Swing, see Figure 3 and follow these steps:

(1) Dig up a Montovani or Percy Faith record and put it on your record player to place you in the slow rhythm the Swing requires. After you have practiced the Swing for a week or so, you may dispense with the music and go at your own particular rate—as long as it is slow and smooth.

(2) Glasses off, stand at ease in the middle of the room, facing a window.

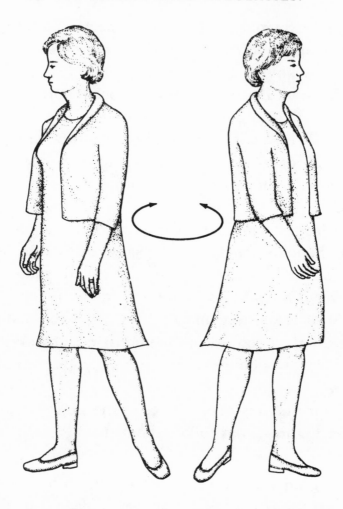

Figure 3.

(3)   Keep your feet parallel and comfortably apart. If
you are quite short, the distance between them
should be about eight inches; if you're a six-
footer, 12 or 14 inches. But don't bother about a
ruler or a yardstick—the best distance between

your feet is the one you find most natural and with which you feel perfectly balanced.

(4) Let your arms hang loosely, and keep your nose pointed straight ahead, as in Sunning.

(5) Now swing your body—head, trunk and all—to the right, putting your weight on your right foot and letting your left heel rise from the floor.

(6) When your shoulders are parallel to the wall that was at your right as you started, swing back to the center, and without pausing, swing on to the left. Your weight will transfer to your left foot, and your right heel will rise.

(7) As you swing, imagine that the top part of the back of your head is extending upward, and that the area around your lower spine is extending backward.

(8) Don't swing too far—you are relaxing not exercising—and don't go beyond the point where your shoulders are parallel to the appropriate wall.

(9) With your head level and your nose pointing straight ahead, let your eyes drift along the lines where the wall meets the ceiling.

(10) After a few swings, lower your eyes to a level just beneath the top of the window, and follow

an imaginary line along the wall. Keep the line straight and uninterrupted, flowing smoothly. This is not as easy as it sounds; you really have to keep your mind on what you are doing.

(11)   When your eyes pass the window, let them gaze out as far as the vista permits—the change of focus will loosen the eye muscles. But keep your vision on the level of that line your eyes have traced across the walls.

(12)   With each few swings, lower or heighten your imaginary line a foot at a time, until you quit.

During the swinging, you will experience an illusion. The window frame will appear to move in a direction opposite to the one in which you are swinging, and so will other nearby objects. Yet things outside the window, such as trees and utility poles, will seem to move along with you. If that does not happen, you have been swinging improperly, holding yourself rigid. The same is true if the swinging makes you dizzy or nauseous—you have been moving rigidly or you have been staring. If you do become dizzy or nauseous, stop for a moment, then resume with the grace and ease that accompany and induce relaxation. (One merit of the Swing is that it breaks the staring habit; another is that it loosens you if you're uptight.)

Ideally, the Long Standing Swing should be performed three times a day—in the morning, sometime during the afternoon, and before bed. Begin with 30 complete swings, and increase the number daily until you are doing 100. If that sounds like a lot, remember that at the rate of 30 swings per minute, a normal enough pace, 100 swings will take a mere three minutes and 20 seconds. That is a small price to pay for a day-long sense of well-being, sound sleep, and better vision.

Perform the Long Standing Swing only as long as it does not bore you—boredom is an enemy of relaxation. If you become bored with the procedure, stop for a few days, or try a variant.

Here's an interesting alternative:

(1)   Swing to the right, in the manner of the Long Standing Swing, and raise your right arm shoulder high, fingers extended.

(2)   When the shoulders parallel the right wall, drop the right arm and raise the left one, fingers also extended, and swing to the left.

(3)   Keep your eyes gazing beyond the fingertips and imagine yourself finger-painting a horizontal black line on the wall.

Except for the raised arms and the "finger-painting," this procedure is identical with that for the Long Standing Swing. Many people, however, find it easier to imagine the lines that way. Because of the raising and lowering of the arms, this routine is something of a calisthenic and rather stimulating, so it is best not to do it at bedtime.

SHORT SWINGS

Older people who find it difficult to stand—as Mrs. H. did —can derive many of the benefits of the Long Standing Swing from similar rhythmic routines called Short Swings. These can be performed sitting down.

One of the best of them, which releases tension of the eye muscles, calls for you to seat yourself comfortably in a straight-backed chair, take off your glasses, and let your arms and hands hang loosely. With your eyes open and your nose pointing straight ahead, turn the upper half of your body from side to side. Your arms should swing with your torso, freely and rhythmically. Your head, of course, must turn with your body. After a few such swings, set your eyes to imagining the same kind of horizontal lines on the wall that are "painted" in the Long Standing Swing.

LAZY EIGHTS

Lazy Eights, of which there are countless variations, consist basically of drawing imaginary Figure Eights easily in the air with your nose. Sounds silly, doesn't it? But Lazy Eights loosen the back of the neck and calm the whole nervous system when you are rigid and tense.

Little Lazy Eights relax tiny muscles in the eyes. Big

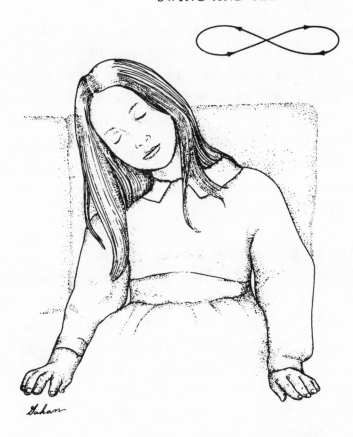

Figure 4.

ones relax the larger muscles and the big Lazy Eights send blood speeding to the brain and throughout the head, neck, and eyes. Big or little, they can be performed any where, anytime, so inconspicuously that no one will notice. I have done Lazy Eights while waiting for an elevator in an office building, in my theater seat during intermission, and while talking on the telephone in my office.

Just close your eyes and draw Eights with your nose

—horizontal Eights, vertical Eights, lop-sided Eights—as you move your head slowly and smoothly. When you tire of Eights, draw pies in the air and cut them into wedges. Draw wagon wheels and put in the spokes. Draw arcs, little and big, in every direction. Sometimes, just move your head slowly and evenly, as if you are moving all the tissues in the head and neck. This requires concentration; imagine that your consciousness is entering your head and neck. See Figure 4.

All the procedures I have thus far described, from Sunning to Lazy Eights, are relaxants, designed to heighten the sensitivity of the entire body, including the eyes. Unlike exercises, which are intended to build and tone muscles and which require little or no thought, sight-training procedures demand concentration. *They must be performed slowly and rhythmically.*

In the following chapters, I shall discuss specific routines for specific eye problems.

HOW TO
CORRECT
EYE DEFECTS

In most refractory defects of the eye, muscular imbalance exists. Some muscles pull too taut, some sag. Each defect distinguishes itself by its own set of maladjustments, and each requires its own remedial approach. Corrective procedures are not difficult, but demand dedication—just reading this book will work no miracles for your eyes.

You must train your eyes to do what you want them to do, and training them requires as much patience as schooling a dog in obedience. Thus, older people frequently achieve better results than young people because they may have more tenacity and more time. But whatever your age, your chances of success are good if you truly want success and work for it.

MYOPIA

One of the most prevalent defects is myopia, or nearsightedness. It generally begins early in life—between the ages of 6 and 10, or sometimes a little later in adolescence. Physically, myopia is the result of an elongation of the eyeballs from front to back. But unless a child is born myopic—a rare occurrence—the cause is usually emotional, the result of some strain: the child is compelled to read before he is ready; or he is bored with school; or as one study showed, he dislikes his teacher, and unknowingly refuses to see the blackboard.

A study of my own indicated that the myopic child is often an extraordinarily well-behaved and obedient child suffering from repression and anxieties of which he is unaware. He shuts out the world which might tempt him to misbehave; he reads with ease, close up, but sees nothing clearly beyond the safety of books. Nevertheless, because there is a definite physical aspect to the defect, myopia often may be corrected without the psychotherapy that its origins would imply was necessary.

To work on myopia, begin with Sunning and Palming for several short periods, and Palming for one longer period. Then stand 14 ordinary dominoes—each having no more than 12 dots—an inch apart at face level. You can array them on a stack of books on a table or desk, on a bookshelf, or on top of a television set.

Sit just far enough away so that the dominoes appear slightly blurred. Take your glasses off—as with all work recommended here—close your eyes, and relax. Your eyes should rest as easily in their sockets as a baby snug and asleep in a cradle.

Now, inhale deeply and slowly. Exhale slowly and

deeply. Open your eyes and let them gently wander around the sides, top, and bottom of the domino farthest to the left. Don't try to see its dots—just look around its boundaries. Try to feel that you are looking from the back of your brain, where visual processing takes place.

Repeat the procedure six times with that domino, then move on to the next one. By the time you have reached the sixth domino, the slight blur with which you began should have disappeared and the domino should stand out vividly.

But if the dots of the domino are not a bright, sharp white, close your eyes and visualize the first domino, mentally intensifying its image as sharper and brighter than you actually saw it. Imprint that image on your memory. Memory is important to vision—we see familiar objects more clearly than unfamiliar ones.

Now open your eyes and while remembering the clearly visualized imagine, let your eyes move again around the sides of the first domino. No matter how you actually see the domino, the memorized and projected image will make it more clearly visible.

Repeat the procedure with the other five dominoes. Each time that one stands out sharply, memorize its pattern and then visualize it with your eyes closed. When all the dominoes look clear to your open eyes, move your chair back six inches and go through the game again. It won't take as long as you may think—half an hour should suffice, but the more time you can devote to it, the better.

The second day, switch from dominoes to playing

cards. Use spades with numbers—no jacks, queens, kings, or aces—because the numbered spades are clearly visible in a simple black-and-white pattern. With clear cellophane tape, fix the cards to a wall at eye level, one inch apart. Sit where they appear slightly blurred and use them as you did the dominoes.

The third day, substitute a calendar with numerals big enough to be read at 10 feet (or closer, if necessary) without glasses, and with only slight blurring. Let your eyes run around the frames of the dates as though they were the sides of the dominoes. You should be able to sit much farther back this time, because of the images imprinted on your mind, and because work with the calendar accustomed your eyes to greater distances.

After eight days of alternating near and far work, break the rank of your dominoes: place some where you can see them perfectly, and another group where they appear slightly blurred. Look back and forth between the dominoes for 10 minutes or so, pausing frequently and concentrating on their peripheries rather than on their patterns. Then resume the regular domino drill for the rest of the time available.

Keep up the routine—dominoes one day, playing cards the next, and the calendar the third—for at least a month. If you wish, in place of the cards and calendar, you may substitute pictures cut from magazines, printed signs, or any other more complicated or more interesting pattern. But always look around the edges of the patterns, not directly at them, and do so with a feather-light gentleness. Interrupt the procedure frequently to change focus.

Play solitaire whenever you can: it induces muscular mobility, and it is devoid of the tensions that exist in competitive card games.

By month's end, anyone with no worse than average myopia should note a considerable improvement in vision; more serious cases will take longer. (In low or moderate myopia, refractive error does not exceed six diopters, a unit of measurement used in optical science. If you do not know the extent of your error, your oculist or optometrist can tell you what it is.)

One client, a co-ed at an upstate New York college, had a single lesson in corrective procedures for myopia and then returned to school to practice the routines on her own. After a month, she found she could read the blackboard without glasses for the first time in all her school years.

Don't quit after a month, though. Continue the routines until you see as well as you want to. Practice whenever you can. In a bus or a train, let your eyes glide lightly over advertising cards, without reading them, as though they were playing cards or calendars. If you look at them for brief periods, it will not matter that they are above eye level. Then shift your eyes to the buttons on the coat of a person across the way, following the periphery of the buttons. You need not feel embarrassment—the motions of your eyes will not be noticeable. If you feel really bold, outline faces and bodies.

HYPEROPIA

Hyperopia, commonly called farsightedness, affects many children and often persists into adulthood. A victim of hyperopia cannot readily focus both eyes on objects close to him, so reading becomes difficult, sometimes causing nausea and headaches. Hyperopia frequently attends a child's poor work in school.

The hyperopic person sees well in the distance but experiences difficulty with close vision. In this anomaly, there appears to be an emotional factor; hyperopia may be another way of handling anxiety. To correct this imbalance, the essential practices are Sunning, Palming, Swinging, and the practice of frequently changing focus from far to near and back again. These procedures must be used, however, in conjunction with several techniques designed specifically to counter hyperopia.

If you want to correct hyperopia in a child, make the procedure a game—if he or she has to practice Sunning, Palming, and the rest like scales on the piano, it won't work. Keep it fun—with the promised reward of better sight, enjoyment in reading, and freedom from headaches and eyestrain.

The first of the specific techniques for correcting hyperopia lends itself well to game playing.

(1) Start with the blank back of a white business card.

(2) Pencil a black dot in its center.

(3) Holding the card in one hand at a comfortable distance, look from one side of it to the other until the dot seems to move left when the eyes look to the right, and vice versa. (This illusion fascinates children.)

(4) After a few minutes of this, add more dots half an inch apart on a horizontal line.

(5) Now, gently shift the eyes from dot to dot, back and forth across the card four times in all.

(6) Then close the eyes, and from memory, visualize the dots. Shift from each to the next as though the eyes were open. Do this, too, four times.

(7) Next, array dots vertically, again half an inch apart. Look up and down the card, four times with your eyes open, four times with them closed.

(8) Take another card and substitute colored dots— in colors that are your favorites—and go through the procedure again.

This card drill may be repeated daily, but especially with a child, make sure that it is done voluntarily. If it is performed as an obligation, it will fail to relax the mind or the eye muscles.

Follow the card routine with this one that makes for easier reading.

(1) Find a book or a sheet or printed matter with plenty of white space between the lines and type that will appear slightly blurred when you hold a page in front of you.

(2) Place the page upside down so you cannot read the text.

(3) Run your eyes gently and slowly around the margins a few times, looking from the back of your head.

(4) Then choose two points at the top corners of the page, and another, such as a box of Kleenex, at a distance within the room.

(5) Shift your eyes from the points on the page to the box and back, several times.

(6) Next, scan the white spaces between the lines, going down the page as though you were reading. By the time you are halfway down, everything will seem clearer. But do not strive for clarity; keep going.

(7) When you reach the bottom, turn the book or sheet right side up, and look along the white space below the first line of type.

(8) Close your eyes now, and from memory paint imaginary white in the space, back and forth.

(9) Open your eyes and scan the spaces beneath the first few lines, envisioning them as being as bright as snow under a brilliant sun. Repeat this several times, alternately closing and opening your eyes.

(10) Then float your eyes back and forth over the lines of type without trying to read them.

(11) Look away, then return to the page. The black of the type will seem blacker, and the white of the spaces whiter than you have ever seen them. The words will stand out sharply.

The first time I tried this routine myself I became so excited over the results that I raced to the telephone to tell Sidney Fields, who had first told me about sight training. But don't let enthusiasm carry you away—devote 15 minutes to the whole procedure, then quit for the day.

In the weeks that follow, gradually reduce the size of the type with which you are practicing until you are able to read the tiny font in which legal advertisements in the newspapers are set.

Alternate the routine with others such as this one: Take a pencil or a colored toothpick and move it from one side of a single word to the other, following the point with your eyes. Do this four times.

Then close your eyes and do it again four times, visualizing the moving point. Repeat the procedure with a dozen words. When you have finished, the whole structure of your eyes will have loosened. (The structure of the eyes tightens when you read something you do not understand, and the tightening results in pressure on your mind and your eyes.)

Another routine for easier reading:

(1)   Place a small calendar at book-reading level, 14 inches from your eyes.

(2)   Choose six dates at random, and shift your eyes from side to side on each in turn without trying to see the dates clearly. (If they are not blurred, move the calendar two inches closer to you.)

(3)   Now close your eyes and visualize one of the numbers.

(4)   Repeat the procedure with the other five numbers, opening and then closing your eyes for each. When you finish, all six numbers will stand out sharply.

The next day, place the calendar 12 inches from you (or 10 if you started with 12), and the following day, two inches closer still.

The whole procedure takes no more than 15 minutes daily, and greatly facilitates close-up reading.

PRESBYOPIA

For average cases of presbyopia, or middle-aged farsightedness (no more than five diopters), the basic corrective routines are identical with those for hyperopia. One significant addition is an emphasis on shifting focus from far to near and back again frequently.

To avoid having to wear bifocal glasses, practice the procedures recommended for myopia. In addition, play solitaire and Ping Pong, and juggle a ball, following its movements with your eyes.

For women, and for men who enjoy it, coarse sewing may prove more appealing. Use the biggest needle, the heaviest thread, and the most loosely woven cloth you can find. After each stitch, raise the needle to arm's length and follow it down and up with your eyes. Or substitute the nail of your forefinger for the needle, keeping your eyes on it as you make great, exaggerated sewing motions, using both hands alternately.

For more advanced presbyopia (more than five diopters), add this routine:

Take a playing card with black numbers and hold it at a comfortable reading level, but so close that the numbers blur slightly. Sit where you can see a picture on the wall some distance away.

Card in hand, outline it with your nose by slight head motions. Then shift your eyes to the picture and outline that.

Alternate between the picture and the card until you

get bored. Then do Lazy Eights for a while, and then return to the picture and the card.

If you can spare 20 minutes, good; but even shorter periods once a day—more often if time permits—will help.

And you might try this one too: Hold a brightly colored ball, or a Christmas tree ornament, or an orange or lemon, and keeping your eyes on it, draw circles in the air with it—small circles and big circles. You will loosen your eye muscles, not to mention your arm muscles, with the simple motions.

Out walking, cast your eyes to the rooftops and treetops, then back to street level, for the changes of focus that serve the same purpose.

CAN CROSSED EYES BE STRAIGHTENED?

Almost as common as the other eye malfunctions that I have been discussing, but far more distressing to parents and children, is strabismus—crossed eyes or squint. Strabismus is the inability of both eyes to look in the same direction at the same time and produce a single image from what they see. It results from a combination of neurological and muscular malfunctions, and is an extreme manifestation of the faulty fusion of vision from which most people suffer in varying minor degrees.

In some cases of squint, double vision results. Since the brain finds this intolerable, it tries to straighten out the double image of the squinting eye. This prolonged action and reaction between the brain and the eye results in a lessening of the acuity of vision in the squinting eye.

Some infants are born with prominent casts, but all children lack proper fusion until they are about 18 months old. In babyhood, apparent strabismus may simply represent a lag in the child's development, for which allowance should be made: the malfunction may go away.

Doctors often recommend surgery to correct strabismus, but surgery has only a cosmetic effect. After surgery, the eyes may appear straight, but they continue to malfunction internally. If surgery is unsuccessful in straightening the appearance of the eyes, a second operation is sometimes performed. But even then, the results may not keep the eyes looking straight permanently.

The approach of sight training to strabismus is to induce nerves and muscles to function properly, so that both eyes will work with equal effectiveness. In strabismus, an eye that turns inward, outward, or in other directions does not do its full share of the job: in some cases, eyes diverge in alternation.

Whether only one eye diverges or the two take turns at it, corrective measures begin with the relaxation techniques—Sunning, Palming, the Long Standing Swing, Lazy Eights. All are to be performed for a week, before you do anything else.

Then, if only one eye is afflicted, and fails to fall into line, add to the Swing in this manner:

Cover the good eye with one hand and, while swinging, extend your free arm. Point with your forefinger in the direction in which the faulty eye cannot readily move. Follow the finger with that eye.

If both eyes are faulty, alternate the drill, first covering one eye, then the other.

Should you experience nausea or dizziness, stop and do Lazy Eights before resuming the finger pointing.

Along with the relaxation techniques—Sunning,

Palming, the Long Swing, and the Lazy Eights—practice crawling on the floor. *Really.* The sight-training
Crawl differs from the crawl of infants before they can
walk—it's more like swimming, and requires you to
keep your belly flat on the floor while you haul yourself
forward, first with your right arm and right leg, then
with your left arm and left leg. Extend each arm as far as
you can, as in the swimmer's Australian crawl. Do the
Crawl at least once a day for at least 10 or 15 minutes. If
it is your child who suffers from strabismus, do the Crawl
with him, so that he will feel it is a game—and so that he
will not quit too soon.

The Crawl was developed by neurologists to promote
the perception of spatial relationships. Despite its seem-
ing improbability, the Crawl is extremely useful in strabismus.

After Crawling, sit in a rocking chair three feet away
from a lighted pole lamp of the kind recommended for
Sunning. Use a bulb of the strength with which you Sun,
and rock back and forth in front of the lamp. Do this at
least once a day.

Then try Handwaving, which is depicted in Figure 5.
It works this way:

(1) Cover your good eye—if only one of your eyes
     diverges—with one hand.

(2) Wave the other hand back and forth straight in
     front of the diverging eye.

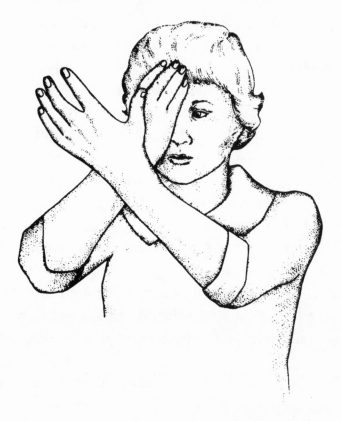

Figure 5.

(3) After several such waves, move your hand off to the right or left, in and out, in the direction the diverging eye refuses to look. Do this four or five times.

(4) Then wave back and forth again, once, and repeat the waves to the left or right, four or five times.

(5) If both eyes diverge, first cover one and wave, then cover the other and wave.

The first week that you do this, restrict yourself to two series of four waves each. Double the waves the second week. The third week, you can do your waves as long as you like. And if you wish, you can start waving a flag, a handkerchief, or a bandanna instead of a bare hand.

After three or four weeks of Handwaving, you will be ready for another technique.

Hold one hand out at arm's length and eye level, with the fingers aligned behind the thumb, as though you were going to do a karate chop. Bring the hand slowly toward you, keeping both eyes on it. When your hand almost touches your nose, turn it so that your palm faces you. Move the hand outward slowly, again keeping your eyes on it. When your hand is out as far as it can go, turn it again to the karate-chop position and bring it toward you. Repeated half a dozen times a day, this technique will help your eyes to converge. See Figure 6, which illustrates the karate-chop position, and Figure 7, in which the hand extends outward, palm toward you.

For children, an excellent procedure involves walking the plank—literally. Set a long plank on three bricks, one at each end and one in the middle. Then have the child walk on it, forwards, backwards, sideways.

For both adults and children, the most important

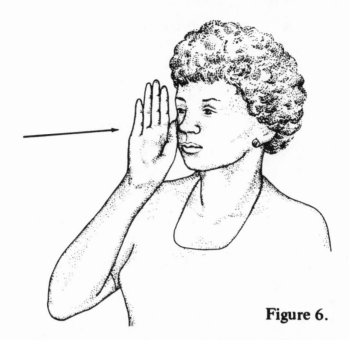

Figure 6.

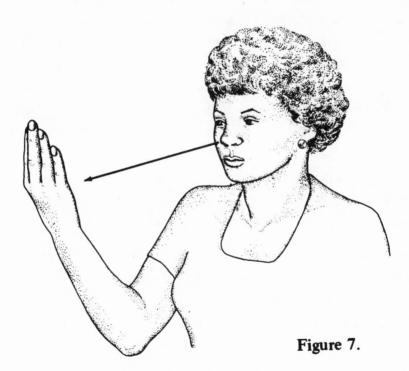

Figure 7.

procedures of all are the fusion techniques described in Chapter "Making Your Eyes See in 3-D". But do not attempt them until you have mastered the corrective measures described in the chapter you are reading now.

A friend of mine who was in her forties used the methods I have detailed, plus the fusion techniques, and obtained a somewhat surprising result. She had long suffered from a paralysis of the eye muscles on one side of her left eye that kept her from moving that eye to the left. The other, relatively good eye was predictably, because of her age, presbyopic.

She Sunned, Palmed, Swung, and Finger-Pointed for some months, as though she was working to correct hyperopia and amblyopia. Gradually, the previously paralyzed muscles got down to work. But, to her great delight, she discovered that she had acquired two bonuses for which she was not prepared.

One bonus was that the hitherto defective eye, unlike its partner, began behaving like a young eye: free of the presbyopia that affected her right eye, it became the better of the two, and permitted her to read with ease.

The second bonus involved an eye injury my friend had suffered, a scratched cornea. Despite the orthodox view that the cornea rarely heals by itself, the injury had healed. Her doctor attributed the phenomenon to the facts that he had cauterized the scratch, and that she had rested for two weeks. But he could not understand why others, treated identically, had not enjoyed the same benefits.

ADDITIONAL
COMMON
PROBLEMS

"Lazy eye" affects almost everyone to some degree, often very slightly. In amblyopia, which is "lazy eye" at its worst, one eye simply does not see so well as the other, although it reveals no defects under examination. Although we commonly refer to the ailment as "lazy eye," this ailment frequently results from psychic suppression of the retinal image. Sometimes the "lazy" eye's vision is spotty, seeing only patches that come in and fade out. But a lazy eye can be roused from its lassitude.

Here's how:

(1)   Cover your willing eye with a patch or a cupped hand and use the unwilling eye alone on dominoes, playing cards, or a calendar. Do this for five minutes at a time in the manner recommended for myopia.

(2)   Uncover the willing eye, and use both eyes to look around the room for change of focus. Glance at the ceiling, the floor, the walls, the pictures, the lamps, the ashtrays, the books.

(3)   Let the eyes glide around the peripheries of the objects, again in the way suggested for correcting myopia.

(4)   From the back of your brain, the main site of vision, direct your attention along an imaginary pathway into the lazy eye. Think through the lazy eye.

(5)   Cover the laggard eye and use the willing eye alone for three minutes or so—but not more than five.

(6)   Now, both eyes uncovered, stand in the middle of the room facing a wall. Hold a pencil, a ruler, or a yardstick vertically at arm's length in front of your nose, narrow edge toward you. (The longer the object the better. A yardstick is preferable, although not absolutely essential.)

(7)   Look up and down the yardstick several times— three or four—then up and down the wall several times. You should remember the image of the yardstick, and see it peripherally as well. If your eyes are working, you will see two yardsticks instead of one while looking at the wall. At

the start, do this procedure for three minutes. Gradually increase the time over a period of several days, and vary your distance from the wall.

(8)   If you do not see two yardsticks while looking at the wall, cover one eye and look beyond the yardstick. Then cover the other eye, and repeat the procedure. The stick, of course, will appear to each eye to be in a different place. Remember the place where the stick appeared for each eye. When you start using both eyes uncovered— while remembering the different places—you should experience the illusion of two yardsticks. If it still eludes you, do Lazy Eights for a while, then return to the yardstick.

When you put down the stick, perform 20 or 30 Long Standing Swings. Use both eyes, and from the back of your brain concentrate on the visual process. Imagine that your eyes are camera lenses, and the film is being developed instantaneously in a darkroom in the rear of the brain.

Also, use the dominoes, playing cards, or calendar, and finish off with Sunning and Palming. Over the weeks, gradually lengthen the time in which you use one eye alone—up to 15 minutes, but no longer—for the eyes must accustom themselves to working together, like a good team of horses. However, never whip either horse.

Keep your mind on the laggard, but work it gently, in a relaxed manner. One good way to do so, as in correcting myopia, is to play solitaire.

ASTIGMATISM

Astigmatism seems to accompany almost every other visual malfunction, and it occurs independently as well. In astigmatism, images blur, and objects you see take on distorted shapes and forms quite different from reality. Astigmatism has its emotional roots, but its physical cause is an irregularity in the curvature of the cornea. Such irregularities result from tension or pressure on the eyelids or the eyeball.

Relax, and the astigmatism diminishes or disappears. To that end, begin with Sunning, Palming, the Long Standing Swing, and Lazy Eights, and follow these with several drills designed to ease shifting of the eyes.

For the first such drill, bend a wire coat hanger into a hoop, and wrap about a dozen inch-long snips of brightly colored tape around the hoop at equal intervals. Hold the hoop broadside before you, at eye level, a foot from your face. Glide your eyes clockwise from one tape marker to the next, with a gentle head motion. Go around the hoop three times.

Close your eyes and, remembering the look of each marker, go around three more times. Repeat the procedure counterclockwise. See Figure 8.

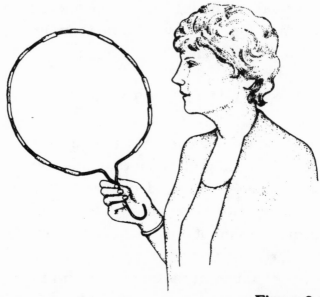

Figure 8.

A second good drill requires a yardstick instead of a coat hanger, and a red pencil or crayon instead of scotch tape.

(1)   Mark off the inches on the yardstick with bold red lines.

(2)   Hold the stick horizontally in front of you, at eye level and arm's length.

(3)   Glide your eyes, from inch to inch, back and forth several times.

(4)   Close your eyes and see the inch marks with your mind.

(5) Open your eyes, and this time, move the stick to the left while your eyes glide right; then to the right, while your eyes glide left. (An optical illusion will seem to heighten the speed of the yardstick.)

(6) Next, hold the yardstick vertically. Eyes open, note the inch marks. Move your head slowly up and down. After a bit of this, move the stick down, while you move your head up, and vice versa. As in all drills described in this book, change focus frequently.

Perform the drills at least once a day, more often if you can. Play solitaire and use dominoes in the way recommended for myopia. In spare moments, wave your arm and follow your hand with your eyes in the technique suggested for stabismus.

SPOTS BEFORE THE EYES

Spots before the eyes, for which the technical term is *muscae volitantes* (flying flies), are common among older people but do occur in the young, especially students. They can annoy—I know, I have had them—but do not let the spots alarm you. Dr. Bates tells of patients who appeared at his office in terror, sometimes late at night, because physicians had advised them that the spots forewarned of glaucoma, blindness, kidney, heart, and liver ailments. It wasn't so. The patients had no eye defects, no fearsome diseases.

The spots are infinitesimally tiny specks floating in the eyes' internal fluids. If they appear, don't look at them, but keep your eyes on bigger, more important things. Don't stare. Don't strain. Sun, Palm, and perform the Long Standing Swing and Lazy Eights. And out, damned spots!

PERIPHERAL VISION

Poor peripheral vision—in which one sees well enough when looking straight ahead, but sees little or nothing at the sides or above or below—is more common than most people realize. Because poor peripheral vision does not manifest itself obviously, victims of the defect may be unaware that they suffer from it.

A friend of mine who was convinced his sight was quite good—he had nothing worse than mild presbyopia—frequently bumped into the door of an over-the-sink kitchen cabinet whenever his wife left it open, as she did much of the time. The resultant rows—he blamed her for leaving the door open, she berated him for his stupidity in not avoiding it—ended only when he removed the door. It was not until I mentioned the possibility of poor peripheral vision to him that he realized the cause of the trouble.

The defect originates in the fact that not all areas of the retina are equally sensitive to light. The defect is especially marked in high myopia and in the serious eye ailment called *retinitis pigmentosa*. Night blindness is a common early symptom of retinitis pigmentosa, a slow degenerative disease of the retina. In advanced cases, only a small portion of the retina functions well, with the result that vision is of the gun-barrel, tube, or tunnel variety. The patient possesses only an exceedingly narrow field of vision, just straight ahead of him.

You can test your own peripheral vision by holding up the palm of one hand about 10 inches in front of your face, and while looking at it, wave the other hand in arm's-length circles. Where you cannot see your waving hand, and a friend with normal vision can see his own waving hand, you lack peripheral vision.

One way to improve the condition is to hold up your two forefingers five inches apart and six inches from your nose. Look at one finger, but keep aware of the other. You will be using central vision on the first, peripheral vision on the second. Shift your eyes back and forth from one to the other—never losing sight of both—and try to take in the whole room, colors and all, at the same time. Then repeat this drill, moving your two fingers six inches apart. You might also try this drill at seven and eight inches.

Another method is to hold up a finger of one hand six inches from your nose and while keeping your eyes on that finger, use your free hand to move a bright-colored ball or a Christmas tree ornament in various directions in which the object disappears beyond your range. When it vanishes, bring it in close, and still looking at your finger, imprint the ball on your memory. When you move the ball outward again, memory will help you see the object where you could not see it before.

Vary these practices with one using candles. To broaden your field of vision horizontally, set four lighted candles on a table at eye level, a few inches apart. Turn out all other lights. Keep all four flames in sight, as you turn your head slowly from side to side; at the same time, fix your central sight or attention at one distant object on each side of the room. If all four candles remain in sight at the far end of each turn, move the candles farther apart until the one at the end opposite the direction of your headturn is out of range. If you are unable to see the farthest candle, try to imagine seeing it. Do this 15 minutes or more each day.

To extend your peripheral vision vertically, use two candles—one candle set high, perhaps on a mantlepiece, the other low—and move your head slowly up and down. As you look at one candle centrally, the other is seen peripherally. To further enlarge the field, keep increasing the distance between the high and the low candles. Here, too, use mental imagery to bring in what is momentarily invisible.

For spare moments, try this one: point a forefinger straight ahead of you at arm's length. Keep your central vision on your fingernail, and slowly swing your other arm above and below the fixed finger in ever widening arcs. Here, too, use mental imagery—that is, *imagine* seeing the ever widening arcs if you cannot *actually* see them.

Or this: while gently looking ahead at an imaginary dot, wave one arm and then the other in wide gestures, as though you were signaling a small plane into a landing. Follow your arm with your eyes.

Or this: hold a bright handkerchief—or a piece of chiffon—at arm's length, and flutter it in great circles, to your sides, above your head, down to your knees. Look straight ahead all the while, but keep the little banner in sight.

NIGHT BLINDNESS

Poor vision at night is a distressing symptom of various eye diseases, retinitis pigmentosa being a good example. Vitamin A deficiency is another cause of night blindness, which may appear as a functional nervous disorder associated with other symptoms of neurosis.

For improving vision at night, apply all the procedures recommended for improving peripheral vision. In addition, practice with dominoes, calendars, and cut-out letters as you would for correcting myopia, but use less light than you would ordinarily. When you find that you can see in rather poor light, diminish the illumination even more—until you can see at night, as well as your friends with good vision can.

MAKING
YOUR EYES
SEE
IN 3-D

Anyone who has almost any common eye defect is likely to suffer from imperfect fusion as well. Imperfect fusion reflects a failure of the eyes to coordinate.

Since our eyes are several inches apart, they see from slightly different angles, like the two lenses of a stereo camera. But the images they transmit to the brain, like the stereo camera's twin slides, must be precise enough to merge into a single perfect picture.

Poor fusion, like most other sight problems, is caused by muscular imbalance and some nerve malfunction. It shows up at its worst in crossed eyes or double vision. In less severe cases, it may produce a slight blurring, headaches, or simply a feeling of strain. Poor fusion hinders depth perception, which is essential in such commonplace activities as driving an automobile. (Airline pilots must have perfect depth perception—hence, perfect fusion—to land a plane.)

Even perfect fusion is not perfect all the time: heavy

drinking, fatigue, emotional upset, or illness will impair it. But if you have never had perfect fusion, to attain it can be an exhilarating experience.

Before you undertake any techniques for acquiring perfect fusion, your eyes must be relaxed; so first Sun, Palm, and do the Long Standing Swing. Do not attempt the fusion techniques at all when you are tired, ill, or under mental strain. When you do undertake them, practice them in the order in which they appear below, progressing from easy to advanced.

THE FIRST TECHNIQUE

(1)   Sit facing a wall about six feet away, and hold a ruler or yardstick vertically, narrow edge forward, a foot from your nose.

(2)   Look up and down the stick three or four times, then up and down the wall the same number of times. As you scan the wall, the stick will seem to become two sticks separated by a space.

(3)   Alternate between stick and wall for three minutes at the start.

(4)   After a few days, lengthen the time and vary the distance from the wall.

Like all procedures for improving fusion—and sight in general—this technique should be practiced slowly, gently, in a state of relaxation.

THE SECOND TECHNIQUE

(1)   Hold a yardstick horizontally, one end three inches from the nose, and the other end pointing toward a wall.

(2)   Glide your eyes along it from the near end to the far end and back, several times. At whatever end you are looking, an illusion of an apex of a V will appear. At any point between the ends, you should see an X.

(3)   If you see a Y instead of a V, your poorer eye is not doing its homework. In that case, cover your better eye and direct the other one back and forth over the stick. Do this several times a day, and you will notice that, when you look along the yardstick with both eyes, the arms of the Y will slide lower and lower until they form a V. You might visualize the V with eyes closed.

If you have no trouble from the start, practice this technique only five or six times a day at first; after a week or so, you may do it longer, letting your comfort be your guide.

THE THIRD TECHNIQUE

(1)   Tie one end of a 20-foot cord to a doorknob or the top of a chair, as illustrated in Figure 9.

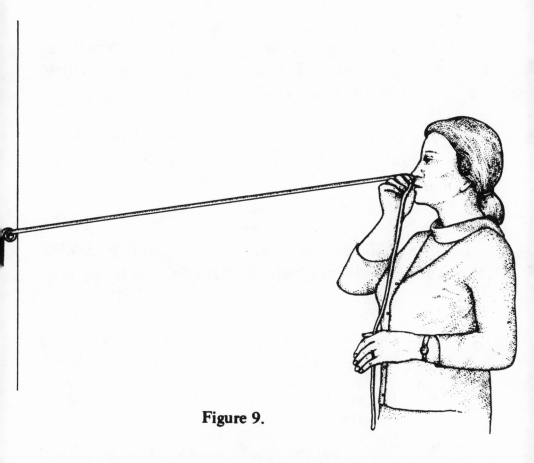

Figure 9.

(2) With head erect and good posture, stand three feet from the knot and hold the cord taut near the tip of your nose.

(3) Shift your weight from leg to leg, let your body sway, and look along the cord to the knot. You should see an illusion of a V.

(4) Move slowly backward, looking along the cord to the knot. Blinking normally, still shift weight, until you have reached the end of your rope. If

the V disappears anywhere along the way, shut
your eyes and visualize it. After several relaxed
openings and closings of the eyes, the V should
appear more vivid.

If you don't see the V at all, or have difficulty with it,
be patient; it will show up. Use this technique several
times daily, three minutes at a time.

For children, this procedure must be varied a bit
because a child usually is unable to perform it on his own,
and needs a parent's help. So, for a child, it is practiced
thus:

(1)   The parent holds one end of the cord. The child
holds the other end to his forehead.

(2)   The child keeps his eyes on the parent's end of
the cord.

(3)   The parent, going slowly backward, lets the cord
out a foot at a time, while moving gently and
rhythmically from side to side. Simultaneously,
the parent moves the cord, keeping it taut,
rhythmically and slowly from side to side and up
and down to six or seven inches above and below
the child's head.

At first, as fusion is established, the child will see less
well with both eyes than he does with either eye sepa-

rately, and will complain of strange feelings in his head. To cope with this, have him practice the reading techniques recommended for hyperopia and the distant-vision techniques recommended for myopia.

After a few days, the child's vision will clear rapidly, and the child will, for the first time, experience truly three-dimensional sight. This takes some getting used to. One young client of mine, after establishing good fusion, saw the world so differently that he was unable to ride his bicycle home, and his mother had to come and get him with the car. His sense of balance had altered radically. But he quickly adapted and was delighted with the result.

"My head opened up," he exclaimed. He was right— a part of his brain was functioning for the first time, giving him a fuller, deeper sense of living.

THE FOURTH TECHNIQUE

(1) Bend a wire coat hanger into a circle, leaving the hook for a handle.

(2) Hold the ring vertically six inches in front of your face, and glide your eyes around it, up the near side, down the far side.

(3) The side you are looking at will appear as a single wire, the opposite side as two wires. This is because you are using central sight on the side you are looking at, and devoting most attention to it.

(On the rest of the ring, you are using peripheral vision.)

(4) Go around the ring four times with your eyes open, then close your eyes and imagine you are seeing the ring as you did with open eyes. Repeat the procedure—four go-rounds with open eyes, then once with closed eyes—half a dozen times. Do this daily.

THE FIFTH TECHNIQUE

(1) Take a piece of cardboard four inches by two inches, lay it down horizontally, and draw a quarter-inch wide red line down its center, from top to bottom. (A piece of tape may be used for the same purpose.) On either side of the line, cut a hole one-half inch in diameter. Place the holes so that their centers are as far apart as the pupils of your eyes—about two inches. See Figure 10.

(2) Sit facing a distant wall. Hold the card close to your eyes and look through the holes at the wall. The red line will appear to become two lines, with a single hole between the lines.

(3) Move the card out to six inches from your nose. There still will be two red lines, but three holes will now appear.

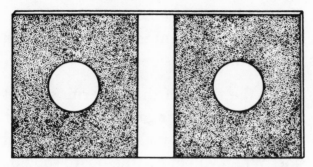

Figure 10.

(4)   Move the card back and forth slowly in an area of six to 14 inches from your nose, continuing for three minutes. Repeat the procedure several times daily.

THE SIXTH TECHNIQUE

This one requires a little carpentry, but the result is worth incalculably more than the effort it requires. An ophthalmologist who tried out the gadget that I have in my office told me enviously that it accomplished its purpose more efficiently than did the thousands of dollars of optical equipment he used toward the same end. But he did not replace his equipment—probably because it looks more impressive to his patients.

(1)   At a lumber yard, get a piece of masonite six feet long and six inches wide.

(2) On one lengthwise edge of the board, saw slits from end to end, three inches apart, and as deep as an ordinary business card.

(3) Along the bases of the slits, run six feet of half-inch, yellow masking tape all along the board on one side, and red masking tape along the other side. When you finish, the board should look like the board in Figure 11.

(4) Now take the blank backs of business cards and draw a line down the precise center of each card from top to bottom. Put a black dot three-quar-

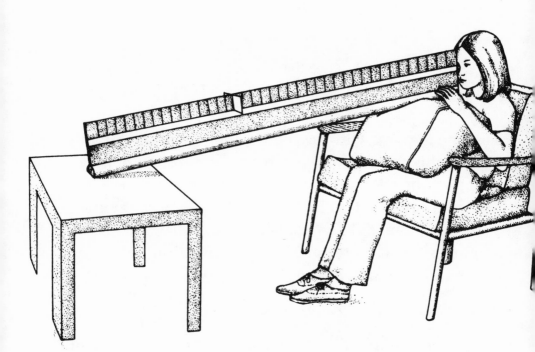

Figure 11.

ters of an inch on either side of the line, centered vertically. (Or simply make a T, as shown in Figure 12.)

(5) Using a child's school compass, make a brightly colored circle around each dot. Each circle should be just large enough to enclose one of two identical Christmas seals, or postage stamps, or geometrical figures such as triangles or squares. See Figure 13.

(6) Center the identical figures on the dots, and paste them down securely.

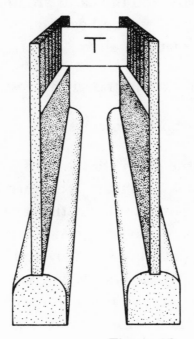

Figure 12.

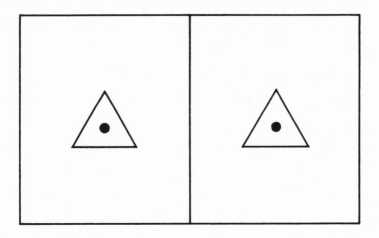

Figure 13.

(7) The board and the cards are now ready for use. Sit down. Rest the board on edge on a table or on the seat of a chair.

(8) Insert a card in the slit nearest to you.

(9) Tilt the board downward.

(10) Hold the end with the card close to your nose and look along the board, using both eyes, to the opposite wall. If both eyes are working well, the board should appear to split in two, creating a path bordered by red and yellow. See Figure 12. If you do not see the path or the colors, one eye is not working. The purpose of using the boards and cards is to make that eye work.

(11) To that end, cover your willing, working eye with one hand or a patch.

(12) Run the other eye back and forth along the board as far as the wall—but keep your eye on the board, not on the wall. Do this several times. Then use both eyes, looking beyond the board again, and remembering what you saw with one eye.

(13) Tilt the board up and down slowly until you see at least patches of pathway. Keep at it for several minutes at a time. While looking at the wall nod your head as if to say Yes. You should eventually see the whole path.

(14) Now to make the two identical pictures on the card merge into one, more or less, look past or through the card toward the wall.

The illusion of two single pictures merging may be blurred at first, especially for those people who have really poor vision. Such individuals may need to tilt the board, or close and open the eyes, or take deep, slow breaths, or imagine the expected merged image. It will take a lot of persistent practice to achieve a single perfect image. Even more important to success in this procedure is a feeling of letting go. But when you have achieved the single perfect image, you will have achieved perfect fusion of your eyes at that particular distance.

If you have difficulty with this technique, interrupt yourself and do Lazy Eights for a while. Blink gently several times. Take some deep breaths. Then go back to the board. Nod your head gently up and down, as you look up and down the near edge of the board, then off to the wall.

When you have achieved perfect fusion at one point, shift the card to the next slit and repeat the procedure. You soon should be able to determine at what distances fusion is poor, and concentrate on those areas.

Because this drill may cause nausea and dizziness at first, it should not be undertaken until you have mastered all those techniques, from the first to the fifth, that precede it. And at the start, you should not practice it for more than 10 minutes a day. You can lengthen the time as your eyes grow accustomed to the work.

You will find the effort worthwhile. For those who take the trouble that this Sixth Technique entails, it will prove to be the most useful of all techniques in correcting poor fusion.

All the corrective procedures for poor fusion require patience. Advance slowly from the easiest to the most difficult. As you practice the techniques, develop and maintain an awareness of both central and peripheral vision simultaneously. Wherever you are, concentrate on using the eye that is responsible for faulty fusion; a patch over the good eye, applied for brief periods in the manner recommended for correcting amblyopia, will help.

YOUR THIRD EYE

A number of Eastern philosophies use centuries-old meditation techniques to link inner and outer vision. You may have seen Indian paintings in which a god or goddess has two normal eyes and a third eye set above them in the middle of the forehead. This represents the integration of what we see with what we understand about our world.

We all have this inner third eye, although many people are not aware of it and so view the world in a flat, two-dimensional way. I have found that people who can learn to visualize with their third eye benefit much more from the 3-D exercises than those who treat them simply as mechanical techniques.

To learn how to visualize with your third or inner eye, let yourself imagine that you too have an extra eye in the middle of your forehead. Imagine a ray of light traveling through that eye straight through your brain to the back of your head. Now, imagine that other rays of light are entering your two actual eyes and converging at the same point in the back of your head. Feel the rays meeting in the occipital lobe at the back of the head, where vision takes place.

As you learn to do this with ease, you will gradually achieve a greater balance in your vision. This can produce a wonderful sense of total well-being, a feeling of being centered that is the goal of all meditation.

All the techniques I have described in the preceding chapters are designed to correct common eye malfunctions. Properly applied, in conjunction with general good visual habits and with relaxing procedures such as Sunning, Palming, and Swinging, they should help to forestall the development of serious eye diseases. Disease generally attacks weakened and vulnerable organs.

But if a serious eye disease does befall you, do not try to cure yourself by this book or by any other book. Go to the best ophthalmologist you can find for diagnosis and treatment. When you are well on the way to recovery, you may find it helpful to practice such relaxing measures as Palming and Lazy Eights. How much you should attempt depends on the nature of the disease. After eye hemorrhages, for example, Palming and Lazy Eights prove efficacious; and once the doctor has told you that the trouble has cleared up, cautious Sunning—beginning with 40-watt bulbs—will help further healing, and will strengthen the blood vessels.

But it is not within the scope of this book—and cannot be—to recommend after-care for each of the many serious diseases that may afflict the eyes.

And now to the question that has been in every reader's mind since he first opened this book: "When can I discard my glasses?" I do not advise you to smash them —as Dr. Bates did—and just go around without them. Take them off wherever you are comfortable without them, at home, in your neighborhood, in a restaurant, and keep them off only so long as you are at ease without them.

At first, those periods of ease may be brief; later, they

should lengthen. Do not expect to see perfectly from the beginning: if you do, you will begin to strain. Just let yourself see what you can see, without trying to diminish blurs or improve them. The results will prove more rewarding than they sound.

I am sometimes asked: "But after I have done the techniques, and strengthened my eyes, won't my muscles tighten up again when I put my glasses back on? I cannot do without them entirely."

The answer is to obtain weaker glasses from time to time. Eventually, you should be able to do without glasses at all, at least for long periods.

In honesty, though, not everyone achieves that happy state simply by practicing the techniques I have described. Vision is nine-tenths mental and only one-tenth physical—its seat is in the brain. How the eye works for and with the brain, how the brain may refuse to see, and how it can be induced to see, are the subjects of the following chapters.

RECENT
CASES OF
INTEREST

In our clinic in New York we have successfully treated many different kinds of vision problems by using the procedures you will learn in the chapters that follow. We always require our clients to have a medical examination first, of course. Based on that diagnosis, we select the exercises that will be most helpful for the particular condition. Many of the clients my staff has worked with have achieved truly remarkable results just by applying themselves diligently to practicing these techniques.

Mrs. C., for example, came to our clinic very unhappy about her double vision. It made her whole life miserable. Everything she looked at had such a vivid shadow that she often could not tell the real object from its shadow. Mrs. C. had a long history of eye problems. For most of her life she had had a "lazy eye" as well as strabismus (crossed eyes). Surgery had corrected the strabismus so that she no longer looked crosseyed, but her vision had not improved until she had started working with an optometrist. He had taught her to use special machines to help her learn to fuse her two eyes. These did somewhat improve the vision in her lazy eye; however, she did not achieve fusion until she began using the relaxation and fusion techniques I taught her. After four months of steady work with me, she was able to see with true binocular, or three-dimensional, vision and was virtually free of the double images that had so disturbed her. This improvement in her sight was accompanied by a marked change in her mood for the better. Not only did the world look clearer to her, but she had also discovered that she could help herself see.

Strabismus can be even more disabling for children than adults. Take the case of J. When he was three or four years old he had two operations to correct his crossed eyes, but this did not improve their fusion. In school he developed reading problems and would not participate in sports. One of our clinic staff, Mrs. Doris Renan, began to work with him when he was ten years old. Like Mrs. C., he was willing to work at the exercises, with the complete cooperation of his parents. To quote J.'s mother, "Our son has made *great* strides in reading this year and is also able to play many sports which he wouldn't play before. He claims he is Number Two soccer player in the school this year because he can finally see the ball!"

Mrs. D. was an unusual case. She was diagnosed as suffering from hyperthyroidism, which brought on an exophthalmic eye condition (bulging eyes). This affected her vision since she had a substantial loss of eye movement as a result, and also proved a constant source of embarrass-

ment. Strangers often stared at her and made rude re-
marks. She consulted doctors, nutritionists, and even ex-
perts in biofeedback, but they could all offer little help or
hope for her condition. After almost five years of search-
ing, Mrs. D. arrived at our clinic and began work with
Mrs. Renan. Let her describe the results in her own
words:

> My condition was an emotional nightmare for a very
> long time. . . . There is no way I can describe or suffi-
> ciently emphasize how much help you have rendered
> by way of the exercises. My own awareness of improve-
> ment was initially in the area of function—that is, I
> realized that looking upwards was becoming possible
> without having to lean my head all the way back to
> compensate for lack of eyeball movement. Gradually I
> also became aware of substantial cosmetic improve-
> ment from the objective comments of others. I have also
> had two opticians indicate recently that in looking at me
> "head on" through my glasses they would not even be
> able to notice the condition.

Another of our staff members, Maria Michal worked
with a middle-aged woman, Mrs. Y., who was diagnosed
as having early macular degeneration in both eyes, which
doctors told her was incurable. After reading the first
edition of this book, she sought us out. The therapist reported that Mrs. Y. applied herself most conscientiously to
the exercises she was taught. After just one week the
morning heaviness she had been feeling in her eyes was
gone. Within eight weeks she could no longer tolerate her

strong glasses, but returned to an old weaker pair. At that point in the eye training, emphasis was switched to drills for the farsightedness she had had before she developed the macular degeneration. After seventeen weekly sessions accompanied by assiduous drilling at home, her doctor examined her and was surprised to find her left eye clear and her right eye with diminished macular involvement. In addition, her distance vision was fine. All she needed was a far weaker prescription for her reading glasses. As a side benefit, Mrs. Y. reported that she was much more relaxed in her demanding job, to the delight of her coworkers. In a year's time she did not need glasses at all, not even at work, and her doctor's report no longer mentioned any macular degeneration in either eye, which he attributed to her having stopped smoking. Mrs. Y. had stopped smoking four years before!

I received a letter telling me of a 50 year old woman who was presented with an ophthalmologist's diagnosis of presbyopia. This is an average type of case without any complications. Generally such aging problems of vision are evident in people starting in their late 30's early 40's and become progressively advanced with age. At first her close point vision appeared blurred at age 45. By 50 she had three changes of glasses for reading, all with stronger lenses. Then the distant vision began to blur and she was prescribed bifocal lenses. Three months ago, a friend presented her with a copy of my book. She practiced the recommended general relaxation techniques and close point drills. Now she reports that the distant vision returned to normal and also that she is able to read at the close point in a good light without any glasses. When fatigued, ill or with inadequate light she needs some reading glasses. Also, she now uses the ones prescribed five years ago, when the first indications of a slight blur occured. This is the usual and expected course of improvement for most people who dilligently apply themselves to doing the drills and learn to read and look without staring or straining.

Cultural differences are no barriers to sight improvement. Another client, Mr. B., came from India to attend Harvard University for one semester at the age of forty-seven. It was a race with macular degeneration, which had been diagnosed two years previously. However, long hours of intensive study quickly took their toll on his vision. After the first four weekly sessions at our clinic with Maria Michal, and dedicated application of the exercises on his part at every available moment, he could study for five or six hours without strain. Previously he had had great difficulty in light and darkness accomodation and was extremely sensitive to glare. Also, he was plagued by seeing lines and flashes before his eyes, so that he depended more and more on his peripheral vision. After four months (seven sessions in New York and four phone calls from Boston), his doctor observed considerable improvement of the left eye. Four months later, when he left for his native India, "land of sun and glare" as he called it, he was certain he had the situation well under control, experiencing constant improvement with every passing week. Most of all, he no longer lived in fear of ultimate blindness.

People of all ages have been able to benefit from these exercises. Mrs. Doris Renan worked with seventy-eight year old twin sisters. Mrs. C. had been told that she would need surgery for advancing cataracts. Her left eye was to be "blanked out" for this purpose. Her sister, Mrs. M., had been diagnosed as having beginning cataracts. Both had been given prescriptions for medication to combat glaucoma. However, they were both opposed to taking any medication on principle. After a year's work in the clinic Mrs. C. wrote the therapist from her vacation resort, "I read more easily and can play cards without my glasses. Also, I can read without my glasses for a short time with the left eye alone—the one that was to have been blanked out." The second twin, Mrs. M., also wrote to say that when she had her most recent eye examination, her eyes were so much stronger that she could wear glasses prescribed for her four years before. A year after this, when their eyes were examined, neither twin was diagnosed as having cataracts or glaucoma.

We find repeatedly that quite severe eye problems respond well when clients are committed to working conscientiously on the techniques they learn and practice at the clinic. Mr. P. came to one of the one-day workshops I give to introduce our approach. He complained of light flashes and also of floaters (small particles) in one eye. Over an eight year period he had had his prescription changed for ever stronger lenses three times. Fortunately, his general health was very good and he did not suffer from headaches, although his work required such close concentration and investment of energy that he had strained his eyes badly. He used this great ability to concentrate to set up a daily routine for himself based on the exercises I recommended. When he came to the clinic several months after the workshop, he no longer had light flashes or floaters. He then told me that, before he attended the workshop, two different ophthamologists had told him part of his retina had been broken off. Yet when he had gone to the eye doctor recently, there was no evidence of any breaks in the retina.

One of my most successful students is a woman I've never met. A friend of my son's gave his mother, an elderly black lady who lives in Georgia, a copy of my book. When he visited her three months later he noticed she was reading without using her glasses. He was overjoyed that his gift had been so helpful to her and he told her so. She looked at him sternly and said, "Your father left me a copy of that book when he died. I've been following those exercises every day for a year now." She could read without glasses and see in the distance for the first time in many years, she said happily, returning his own copy of the book to him.

Not everyone who uses the approach presented in this book will improve as readily as that lady. What distinguishes her and most of the other people you've met in this chapter is their spirit. They are conscientious without being overly compulsive; they have the ability to concentrate on each technique to get full benefit from it. When people write in to tell me they have followed the exercises to the letter and still haven't improved their vision, I suggest that they spend time first just learning to relax and focus their attention. The new chapter on "The Wisdom of the East" gives additional ways to do just that.

I had a patient, in my work as a Gestalt therapist, who suffered from extremely blurred vision. She had also had a breakdown accompanied by hallucinations. It was impossible for her to hold a job, let alone concentrate on eye exercises, even under my direct guidance. For two years I did not attempt to treat her eye problems. I simply taught her the different relaxation techniques found in this book, as part of her total therapy. Gradually she was more and more able to Palm and do the Swings on her own and even to meditate every day. At the end of two years of psychotherapy, she could function in her work again and also see clearly without glasses.

Techniques such as Palming and Swinging, self massage and yoga breathing are all basic to alleviating whatever vision problems you may have. In fact they are the cornerstone of healthy sight from the time your children are small. If children would learn these techniques just as they learn to brush their teeth, and make them part of their daily routine, they might never need to wear eyeglasses at all.

THE
WISDOM
OF THE
EAST

As our window on China has opened wider in the past few years, we have learned that the Chinese place great emphasis on eye training in their educational system. In a nation where ninety-nine percent of the young people were once afflicted with myopia (near- or short-sightedness), today it is said that fewer than one percent need to wear eyeglasses for this condition. Other eye problems have shown a similarly dramatic decrease. How has this come about?

It seems that Chinese schoolchildren are led through a series of eye exercises by their teachers for twenty minutes every morning and afternoon. These simple exercises, done regularly from childhood, appear to have played a major part in improving the vision of Chinese youth. Healthier nutritional habits and more humane child rearing practices have also contributed to the improved eyesight of so many Chinese children. Certainly, such exercises will be more successful when a person feels healthy and relaxed.

Our eyes need an unhindered flow of blood and oxygen to function at their best. Often, however, we slow down this flow by tensing our facial and eye muscles unconsciously. Applying pressure to specific areas of the face, as Chinese schoolchildren learn to do, helps stimulate circulation and relieve tension in the eyes. To practice the eye exercises used by the Chinese, look at the chart and follow these step by step directions:

(1) Sit in a straight-backed chair in a comfortable position. Your feet should be flat on the floor and your body should feel supported by the chair.

(2) Place the ball of the index finger of each hand on the bony ridge above the outer corner of your eyes. Rotate your fingers gently so that the skin moves over the bone. Use just enough pressure to feel the bone underneath. Do this with your eyes closed for a slow count of eight. The area may be tender because of tension, but the sensation should be pleasant. You will find that the pain usually lessens as you continue to apply gentle pressure in a rotary motion.

(3) Now place the balls of your index fingers on the same bony ridge, but this time above the inner corner of your eyes, near your nose. Rotate your fingers for a slow count of eight.

(4) Move the balls of your fingers down slightly so that they rest just under the bony ridge at the

EYE EXERCISES

FROM THE PEOPLE'S REPUBLIC OF CHINA

1. Keep eyes closed while doing the exercises.
2. Fingernails should be short and hands clean.
3. Massage lightly and slowly until the area becomes a little bit sore; do not use excessive pressure.
4. Do eye exercises twice a day - once in the morning and once in the afternoon - while sitting with elbows resting on table.

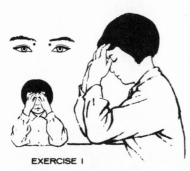

EXERCISE I

Use thumbs to massage inside eyebrow corners with other fingers slightly curled against forehead. (8 times)

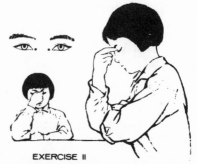

EXERCISE II

Use thumb and index finger to massage nose bridge. Press downward and then upward. (8 times)

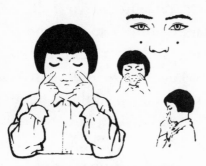

EXERCISE III

With thumbs on lower jawbone, place index fingers and middle fingers together against both sides of nose near nostrils. Then lower middle fingers and massage the cheeks where the index fingers remain. (8 times)

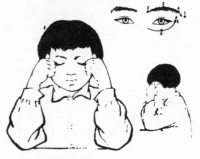

EXERCISE IV

With fingers curled under and thumbs on each side of forehead, use the sides of the index fingers to rub outward following the diagram pattern: 2-3-4-6-5. (8 times)

© 1976

PRICE: $1.00   PUBLISHED BY U.S.-CHINA PEOPLES FRIENDSHIP ASSOCIATION EAST BAY, P.O. BOX 9317, BERKELEY, CA 94709   PRINTED BY THE ALBANY PRESS inner part of the eye socket. This area is called the canthus. Rotate the skin here as you did before, or try something new. Press gently against the bone with your fingers and release, press and release, at least eight times. Experiment to find out which kind of pressure works best for you in the canthus. I like to use both motions, the rotation and the press, myself.

(5) Next, find the hollows under your cheekbones. Press the balls of your fingers into the center of each hollow. Press and release for a count of eight, then try rotating your fingers for a count of eight. If this area, where the sinus cavities are located, is very tender you may want to return to it when you have completed the whole sequence, for a second massage.

(6) Finally, return to the bony ridge over the eyes. Starting at the outer corners near the ears again, slowly rotate your fingers in tiny circles over the whole ridge until you reach the inner corner above the nose. Do this several times to release the tension there.

Like the Chinese school children, spend twenty minutes twice a day on these eye exercises to gain maximum benefit from them. They will give you a wonderful new sense of well being as they bring nourishment to your eyes. If you suffer from tension headaches or sinusitis, you may enjoy continuing with a full head massage to stimulate circulation throughout the skull.

HEAD MASSAGE

Many people develop tension and pain in the temporomandibular joint (TMJ), which connects the jaw to the rest of the skull. To find the TMJ, place your fingers on your cheeks directly in front of the middle of the ear. As you move your jaw from side to side you will feel the joint move. Massage it gently in a circular motion for a count of eight, then press and release for another count of eight.

Continue moving your fingers down the sides of your face, along the jaw line under the earlobes. This is frequently a tender spot. Rotate your fingers for a slow count of eight. If the area is particularly tender, try pressing and releasing as well. The tenderness is usually a sign that circulation is poor, often because of excessive tension.

Follow the line of the skull from your ears around the back of your head until your fingers meet above the spine. The muscles that join the head and neck may be quite tense. This is a good area to massage before you begin Sunning, or using light, to get the greatest benefit from it.

Now try using your fists to massage the rest of your head, including your hairline on the forehead. Use your fists gently, but vigorously enough to increase circulation over your whole head. You should feel revitalized as you do this. For an extra treat ask someone else to massage your head for you. Relax and enjoy as your tension drains away. Try to massage your head twice a day, especially if you find many tender points as you apply pressure.

Some people suffer from chronic headaches that can become incapacitating even though there is no medical cause to be found. They may need a deeper kind of massage than I have outlined here. Most large cities have practitioners trained in structural integration approaches such as Rolfing or the Feldenkreis method, both of which can help improve circulation in the head as well as the rest of the body.

THE BREATH OF LIFE

China is not the only eastern country that has given us ways to improve our vision. For years I have incorporated variations of Yoga breathing from India into my sight training program. As I have stressed, our eyes need nourishment in the form of blood and oxygen. Increasing the oxygen supply in the body is vital to our overall health as well. Yoga breathing is a simple, yet powerful, exercise that helps us begin and end each day with greater clarity and peace of mind. Here is how to do it.

(1)   Sit or stand in a comfortable position, your back straight but relaxed. Breathe in slowly to the count of six, letting the air move into your head, then down through your body as far into the pelvic region as it will go without being forced.

Practice and concentration will gradually produce deeper breathing, so be patient with yourself if your breaths are shallow at first.

(2)   Hold for a count of three, then exhale slowly to
the count of six. As the air rises out of your pelvis
and lungs into your head, say "O-o-o-om-m-m"
to accompany its exit through your nostrils and
mouth. You will hear a pleasant vibration inside
your head as you do this. OM is one of the most
ancient sounds in human speech, and its soothing and revitalizing effect seems to be universal.

Begin by inhaling and exhaling for a slow count of six,
then see if you can slow your breathing down to a count
of ten or twelve for each inhale and exhale. This will allow
you to increase the amount of air you are drawing in and
expelling with each breath.

Once you feel comfortable with this exercise, try a
second breathing technique that aids circulation and
gently massages the muscles throughout the body.

(1)   Hold your left index finger gently against your
left nostril so that the air enters through your
right nostril only. Concentrate on letting the
flow of air move first into your head, then down
into your body as far as the pelvis and groin.

(2)   Open your left nostril and place your right index
finger against the right nostril to close it. As you

slowly exhale, be aware of the air flowing up through your body into your head and out the left nostril. Inhale and exhale should each take about five seconds.

(3)   Inhale through the left nostril and out through the right, reversing the above procedure. Remember, do not force the air in or out. Rather, focus your attention on achieving a slow, natural flow.

All of the techniques described in this chapter should be used along with Palming and Swinging on a daily basis, no matter what other exercises you do for your particular eye problems. They should become part of your total exercise plan for life. The energy and sense of health you will gain as your circulation improves and your body and mind become more relaxed and centered, will soon convince you that the time spent learning these new techniques has been time well spent.

HOW
AND WHY
THE EYE
CAN SEE

Except for the brain that it serves, the eye is the most intricately and elegantly engineered of human organs. But how it evolved remains a mystery that science may never solve.

A possible clue to the origin of the eye lies in the fact that single-cell creatures, who live in the sea where all life presumably began, possess areas called eyespots that are sensitive to light. These areas are not true eyes, for they can merely distinguish between light and darkness. However, these eyespots permit the tiny organisms to find the light they need for manufacturing energy, and enable them to evade light when it is destructively strong. Scientists speculate that over millions of years eyespots developed into primitive eyes that facilitated the emergence of life from the sea onto dry land.

Whether primitive eyes stimulated the growth of a brain because they required a central station to receive and act on their messages, or whether the brain evolved first and then stimulated the growth of eyes, no one knows. In any case, the human brain, very early in its fetal development, projects the optic nerve that links the brain and the eye and transmits signals from eye to brain.

However eyes evolved, nature has been richly inventive in devising them and frugal in distributing them. Most creatures—insects, fish, animals, and man—have only a pair a piece, although there are such exceptions as eight-eyed spiders and one-eyed crustaceans. But the design, placement, and keenness of the eyes vary greatly to suit their possessors' needs.

The dragonfly, living on smaller insects, must be able to spot a gnat anywhere in its vicinity. Thus nature, instead of giving the dragonfly movable eyes like man's, which see in one direction at a time, has provided it with eyes which look every which way at once without moving. In some varieties of dragonfly, each eye has as many as 28,000 separate hexagonal facets, with no two facets focused in precisely the same way. Each facet sees a tiny part of the whole picture.

A tiny tropical fish called *anableps* finds its food on the water's surface, but has to keep watch for bigger, deeper-swimming fish that count anableps as part of their diet. Anableps enjoy bifocal eyes, exactly like bifocal spectacles; the upper halves of its eyes see clearly on the surface, the lower halves are sharpest underwater.

An eagle flying at 1,000 feet can spot a rabbit in deep grass, and a rabbit—fortunately for it—has eyes that allow it to see in all directions at once. It can nibble the grass and see all around it without ever turning its head.

The cat, to enable it to hunt by night, has eyes equipped with a great quantity of cells that are sensitive to minimal light. A cat can see in light so faint that man, primarily a daytime animal, would call it darkness.

Men have always been fascinated by their own eyes. The ancients understood ocular structure well enough to permit them to operate on the eye; the Babylonians had eye surgeons who were made to suffer amputation of a hand if an operation failed; and in India, cataract lenses were being cut out a thousand years before the Christian era.

In modern times, the eye is inevitably compared to a camera, but that is a little like comparing a space ship to a model T Ford. An inch-long spherical sac, the eye takes hundreds of millions of pictures a year, shifts focus instantaneously, and exposes the same film over and over. It is equipped with an automatic lens cap—the eyelid—that is lined with a fine membrane called the conjunctiva, which extends over the eyeball as well, linking eyeball and eyelid.

The eyeball—the spherical sac—rests on a cushion of fat and fibrous tissue in a conical socket formed by the bones of the skull. It is anchored to the bony orbit of the skull by six muscles that (1) change the shape of the eyeball for change of focus, (2) control its movements and, (3) normally, keep both eyes synchronized. Because these muscles are outside the sac, they are called extrinsic muscles; parts of these extrinsic muscles respond to conscious

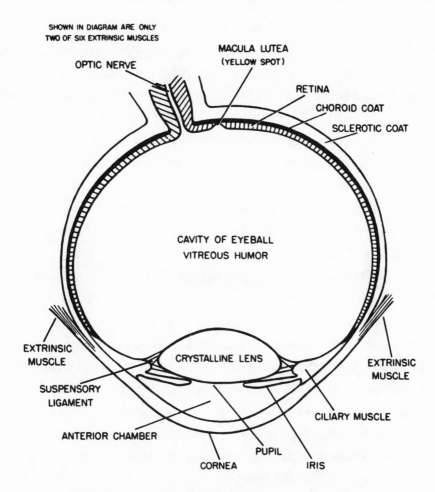

SHOWN IN DIAGRAM ARE ONLY
TWO OF SIX EXTRINSIC MUSCLES

OPTIC NERVE

MACULA LUTEA
(YELLOW SPOT)

RETINA

CHOROID COAT

SCLEROTIC COAT

CAVITY OF EYEBALL
VITREOUS HUMOR

EXTRINSIC
MUSCLE

CRYSTALLINE LENS

EXTRINSIC
MUSCLE

SUSPENSORY
LIGAMENT

CILIARY MUSCLE

ANTERIOR CHAMBER

PUPIL

CORNEA   IRIS

VERTICAL SECTION THROUGH EYEBALL

Figure 14.

commands from us—permitting us, for example, to roll
our eyes—but other parts function automatically, without
conscious command from us, so long as they are not constricted by nervous tension.

The eyeball itself is a kind of Chinese box of three shells or tunics, as optical science calls them, fitted one within another. The outermost is the sclera—the white of the eye—which is a tough, fibrous membrane of numerous layers, any one of which can still function if those in front of it are scratched or otherwise damaged. Five-sixths of the sclera is opaque; but set into it like a crystal in a watch is a five-layered window, the cornea, which opens on the world. The sclera embraces the whole eyeball, and at its rear has a door for the optic nerve that connects the eye to the brain.

The second tunic, the uvea (choroid), gets its name from the Latin *uva* for grape because of its shape. It is a three-part device with widely differing functions. At its front, just behind the cornea, is the iris, a curtain with an aperture, the pupil, at its center. The iris works like the diaphragm of a camera: two tiny sets of muscles within it contract or dilate the pupil to regulate the amount of light the eye admits. But most of the uvea is made up of the choroid, a dark, opaque, multilayered membrane full of blood vessels. These blood vessels nourish the retina—the eye's film—in the third and innermost tunic and pipe away its waste. The choroid also performs the function that the dark chamber performs in a camera.

Toward the front of the eyeball, the choroid thickens into a set of involuntary ciliary muscles called the ciliary body, the exact purpose of which is a matter of dispute. Nonetheless, it is widely believed to work in conjunction with the crystalline lens. This crystalline lens, made up of layers of transparent tissue, floats behind the iris, in a clear fluid called the aqueous humor which is found in the anterior chamber. This fluid fills the spaces under the cornea and around the iris, keeping them in shape and in place.

But without its third tunic, the retina, the eye would remain an unloaded camera. The expanded termination of the optic nerve, the retina, is named from the Latin word *rete* for net because it resembles a pinkish net. Shaped like a tiny curved cinema screen, it is a paper-thin membrane of 10 layers protected by a whitish, jelly-like substance called the vitreous. On its ninth layer, in a space no bigger than an ordinary U.S. postage stamp, the retina crowds between 125 and 150 million photoreceptors—cells sensitive to light.

Some 7 million of these photoreceptors are cones, designed to provide acute vision in bright light; they make it possible to discern color, size, shape, and detail. The cones are largely concentrated in a small part of the retina called the macula lutea ("yellow spot"). The most sensitive of the cones, those that seek out rather than merely respond to light, center in the fovea ("pit"), a miniscule dimple in the macula lutea. We see best looking straight ahead at objects that register on the cones of the macula.

The other millions of photoreceptors are rods. These are scattered over the retina, with the greatest number near the retina's outer edges. The rods provide sight at night, when the cones of the macula and the fovea rest insensitive in darkness. By day or by night, they give us peripheral vision. Where the optic nerve enters the eye-ball from the brain, there are neither rods nor cones, and there the retina has a blind spot.

How this complex mechanism of cornea, iris, pupil, lens, and retina—and a great deal more that I have omitted for the sake of simplification—functions remained a mystery to men long after they understood the physical structure of the eye. The Greeks of the classical age, who knew a good deal about the eye, reasoned that vision was possible because the eyes emanated rays of light which illumined and made visible whatever they touched. (These Greek scientists failed to answer the objection of Aristotle, who wanted to know why, if the eyes gave off light, they could not see in the dark.)

The truth did not begin to emerge until relatively modern times, about 350 years ago, when a German Jesuit, Christopher Schreiner, demonstrated that light enters the eye. Rays of light are collected and initially refracted by the cornea. The iris regulates the intensity of the rays as they pass through the pupil. The light rays fall on the crystalline lens, which brings them into sharper focus and projects them on the retina. (But as Dr. Bates proved the eye can function without the lens.) The retina does not "see," however. It converts the light it receives into energy, and transmits that energy in the form of electrical signals along the optic nerve and other nerve pathways to the brain. It is the brain that translates the signals into images and does our actual seeing for us.

Aldous Huxley, who credited his own recovery from

near-blindness by visual training in the Bates method, summed up the phenomenon of sight in *The Art of Seeing:* "The eyes provide us . . . with the raw materials of sight. The mind takes these raw materials and works them up into the finished product, normal vision of external objects."

If the brain fails to "work up" the raw materials efficiently—as it often does—the eyes may function perfectly yet the "finished product" will prove unsatisfactory. The fault is not one of vision but of perception—of the ability to understand what one is looking at. An infant in a crib may look at a window box and "see" it clearly, but the tot will not perceive that object is a window box because it has had no experience with window boxes. Thus, its brain cannot interpret a "window box" yet. If the child is normal, however, it will learn to perceive that window box and all other window boxes by the time it toddles.

But the inability to perceive is not uncommon in older children, and in adults. In its most serious forms, the inability results from a malfunction of the brain, a snafu in communication between the area that receives the retina's signals and the area that interprets them. It may be organic, it may be caused by emotion—notably shock or fear or anger—and in children it may be a symptom of lagging development. Children who are slow to read and to learn frequently suffer from perceptual disabilities, for which various therapies have been devised.

In its milder manifestations where no brain malfunction exists, poor perception may simply reflect a kind of withdrawal from the world, a desire to avoid the unpleasant and the bothersome. Oedipus blinded himself to shut out what he could not bear to see. Less dramatically, a motorist pausing at a gas station looks at his tires and notes only that they are properly inflated, but the youth who fills the gasoline tank detects, almost without thought, that the left front tire is dangerously worn on the inside because of a wheel misalignment. The motorist did not perceive that because he was mentally evading trouble and expense; the youth did perceive it because faulty tires are part of his livelihood.

Perception is essential to good vision; and where there is a will to see better, there is a way to improve perception—by enlisting memory and visualization, which is the creation of mental images. We see and perceive best the things we know, because their images are familiar to the eye. The signals they impel are familiar to the brain, requiring virtually no effort for interpretation. Just the other day, I read in the New York *Times* of a vacationing college student who discovered dinosaur tracks in a rock outside the factory where his father worked in New York's Rockland County. Many thousands of people had seen the tracks without ever perceiving them, because dinosaur tracks were an unfamiliar sight. But the student perceived them immediately because he had seen dinosaur tracks before, and was thus primed to see more.

Even where we want to see, the new and the

strange cause trouble. The eyes stare to take in the unusual images and the brain strains to interpret them—that is why an hour of sightseeing can prove more wearisome than a day of routine work. If the unfamiliar becomes familiar, however, the brain will perceive and interpret it, even when the eyes themselves function poorly.

Dr. Bates used this phenomenon to improve the sight of a physician who had worn glasses for 40 years, and without them, could not see the big C on the standard eye chart at 20 feet. Though the C was of course black, he saw it as gray, with a gray cloud obscuring its opening. Bates assured him that the letter was perfectly black, the opening perfectly white, and showed it to him up close. When the chart was moved back to the 20-foot distance, the physician remembered what it had looked like up close, visualized its black and white, and saw the letter sharply without glasses. This procedure was repeated down the chart. Within a few minutes, the physician was reading at 20 feet the line that most people see clearly only at 15 feet. A year later, the physician demonstrated to Dr. Bates that he had achieved perfect sight, both close up and at a distance: he could read the smallest type in his newspaper, and distinguish people in automobiles across the Hudson River.

Memory and visualization are essentials in improving sight and perception. But memory functions best when we are relaxed. Everyone has strained to recall a name "on the tip of his tongue," only to have it pop up in the mind later—when the straining has stopped. The relaxing procedures described earlier in this book will improve memory, and with it, vision.

But many people claim to find it difficult or impossible to visualize. If you are one of them, try this:

Face a blank wall, look at it and run your hands over it. Then close your eyes and continue to feel it. Do this three or four times a day, for 10 or 15 minutes, for several days.

Then make a geometric figure—a circle, a square, a triangle—out of a piece of thick cardboard or corrugated paper, three or four inches square, and fix it to the wall with tape. Look at it, feel it. Then close your eyes and move your fingers over the figure, experiencing its shape, texture, and size.

After a few days, when you have become thoroughly familiar with it, substitute cut-out letters and numbers, close your eyes, and familiarize yourself with their feel and shape and size. Then, with eyes still closed, visualize the cut-outs.

When you find your ability to do so improving, take two identical pictures of an animal or a flower—you can cut them from a magazine—and place one several feet in front of you. Hold the other. Run your fingers over the one you are holding. Close your eyes. Project the image of the picture in your hand onto the one farther away. Open your eyes slightly and continue to project the image. Repeat this for brief periods over several days.

For a change, practice this technique:

(1)   Close your eyes and imagine yourself facing a blank wall.

(2)   Then imagine you have a bucket of paint of one of your favorite colors, and a big brush in your hand. Paint with broad strokes, up and down, across, or in patterns. Do it only as long as you feel like it—then quit and differentiate in your mind between the painted and unpainted portions of the wall.

(3)   Now imagine another bucket of paint, of a different color, and a finer brush. Working where you have previously painted, use the small brush and the new paint to make circles—big ones and little ones—and oblongs of varied dimensions. Then paint them out with the first imaginary paint you applied.

(4)   Next, go back to the second color. Paint squares, and take care to get the corners sharp. Paint squares all over the wall—lengthen the handle of the brush to reach high. When the wall is covered, paint out your squares and paint in tri-

angles of varying size, again taking care with the corners.

If all this sounds somewhat irrational, there is method in this madness. The letters of the alphabet—the raw materials of reading—are based on circles, squares, triangles. Apart from the alphabet, there are circles, squares, and triangles all about us. When we learn to visualize them with our eyes closed, we are better able to perceive them with our eyes open.

Ninety-five percent of the clients with whom I have worked have found these techniques effective. Readers who try them on their own will need patience and persistence and concentration. But in the end, you will discover that the eyes have far greater powers than you ever gave them credit for.

The five percent who are not able to visualize after practicing these procedures should keep in mind the fact that one is able to perceive images while dreaming. It may be a deep-seated need not to see some aspect of yourself which prevents the ability to visualize. Be kind and patient with yourself.

THE EYES,
THE BODY,
AND
PSYCHOTHERAPY

On a few occasions earlier in this book I have referred to us as "having eyes." It was a convenient phrase, but it was inexact. We do not "have" eyes or hearts or livers or brains—we *are* eyes and hearts and liver and brains and many other things, as well. All are interdependent and coordinated in single organisms—ourselves—in which the whole is greater than and different from the sum of the parts.

Because of this interdependence of our many components, good eyesight—or rather, the health of our eyes— is fundamentally related to the health of our minds, to our psychic selves. In this particular discussion, diseases of the eye due to accidents, foreign bodies, infections, etc., are obviously excluded. When something goes wrong with our eyes, or any other part of the body, it is not an isolated phenomenon. No malfunction is.

Every difficulty reflects trouble elsewhere, such as a deep anxiety, or a sense of personal inadequacy, a feeling of inability to cope with the world. And two people with identical hidden fears—fears that they hide even from themselves—may develop quite different physical failings, for each of us chooses subconsciously his own way of distracting attention—his own and others'—from his problem.

The individual who becomes nearsighted, or farsighted, or astigmatic, or who has a crossed eye or a lazy eye or strained eyes, is expressing his difficulty in functioning as a whole person. He generally feels he dare not see or be seen; or he compensates for his sense of inferiority by straining and staring so hard that he eventually distorts the structures of the eye and impairs its functioning.

In myopia—nearsightedness—the eyeball elongates because a myopic individual is usually, without conscious knowledge, pushing out and deforming his eyes. This explanation of myopia, which applies also to hyperopia, is my own. Theories that relate myopia and hyperopia to inheritance, poor nutrition, bad reading habits, and other abuses of the eyes have been disproved statistically in two separate research studies (one of which I conducted, the other in which I had no part).

I have found that when ordinary sight-training techniques fail it is because the person involved does not feel safe enough to abandon the defenses he has erected. This was demonstrated rather remarkably in the case of one of my sight-training clients, the renowned psychiatrist and philosopher, Fritz (Dr. Frederick S.) Perls.

A refugee from the Nazis, Perls seemed half Santa Claus and half Biblical prophet. When he came to me in Florida for sight-training, he was 62 years old and was suffering from myopia in the right eye, and amblyopia in the left eye, which was badly inflamed and losing vision. After five lessons, he began to have flashes of good vision. The improvement terrified him, for despite his profession and his appearance of serenity, he was at times a deeply troubled man. He relapsed into myopia, as into a hiding place. The remissions from myopia were physically uncomfortable to him.

It was at Dr. Perls' suggestion that, in what I believe was an unprecedented approach, we combined psychotherapy and ordinary sight-training techniques. Simultaneously, Dr. Perls' vision improved, and he conquered the habits that had distressed him. When he died at age 77, he enjoyed normal sight.

I am convinced that the application of psychotherapy, as refined by Dr. Perls, represented a notable advance toward improving vision in cases where tensions are so deep-seated that sight-training techniques alone fail to produce permanent success.

The innovation was subjected to one of its most severe tests—and it has had many—by a young woman client whose eyes were physically perfect but who could not see. She had been raised in a prim Southern household where her mother had required her to read the Bible for three hours daily. In resentment, the young woman took refuge in blindness. When psychotherapy brought her to

the point of expressing her anger at her mother's rigor—
an anger she had not acknowledged even to herself—she
regained her sight.

In both cases—Dr. Perls' and the young woman's—
the psychotherapy was of the school known as "Gestalt,"
and of the form of Gestalt developed by Dr. Perls. (Gestalt
is untranslatable from the German, so the name has stuck
in English in preference to such imperfect synonyms as
"constellation" and "set-up."

I would like to suggest some additional ways you can
help yourself improve your own eyesight, based on the
theories of Gestalt psychotherapy. Many people have
written to tell me they find it almost impossible to concentrate and relax as I ask you to do throughout this book.
They feel too restless or are full of unhappy feelings that
take up much of their energy.

If you are too restless to Palm, for example, you may
be holding back a great deal of unexpressed emotion over
past or present injuries and injustices. You can help yourself release this restlessness—and feel much better in general—by standing up and letting your whole body shake.
Don't force it, just let the restlessness come out in your
body and especially your hands. Shake them and, at the
same time, sigh or groan or cry, whatever you feel most
like doing at the moment. As you learn to let your body
express its pent-up emotions, you will experience longer
and longer periods of inner calm during which you will be
able to work at the exercises in this book.

When you can allow yourself to live more comforta-

bly in the world, you will find your field of vision expand-
ing both figuratively and literally. This experiment may
help you understand better what I mean. Right now, become conscious of the chair you are sitting in as you read.
Feel the weight of your body settling into the chair seat.
Feel your feet resting on the floor, held there securely by
gravity. Breathe normally. Notice how the chair and floor
support you. You don't need to do a thing to keep from
flying apart—the natural force of gravity is always here to
hold you together although you may not always be aware
of it.

Expand your field of vision to become aware of it
now. Slowly and deliberately let gravity pull your shoulders down into a more relaxed position. Feel your strong
pelvic bones, which hold your body upright, in contact
with the chair seat. All of your senses should begin to
awaken as you perform this exercise. Your whole pelvic
region between the waist and the knees will seem more
alive as you focus your attention on it. Feel the weight of
your feet on the floor. Your legs may suddenly seem very
heavy, then begin to tingle with energy.

Raise your eyes and look around you. Don't try to see
anything in detail. Just be aware of color and motion. Use
your senses of smell and hearing. Let aromas and sounds
come into your olfactory organs and ears without straining for them or shutting them out. Most of all, use your
sense of touch. Let one hand stroke the other. Many people find it very comforting to do this with their hands over
their heart, as if they were holding and stroking a small

baby. As you do this, you may feel your whole body relaxing. Try to imagine that you are a child being cared for and consoled for your hurts. Let your mind bathe in this pleasant experience for as long as you can. Look around yourself again, when you feel ready. People often report that colors appear brighter and objects have greater clarity after this exercise.

Most of us do not allow our organs to function at their full potential. Because we link them to certain painful sights or sounds, for example, we try to avoid such experiences by limiting our vision or hearing. Gradually the world becomes dead for us as we cut off our senses and emotions. We do not have to continue crippling ourselves, however, as I have shown through the simple experiment presented here.

Whether your sight problems are of the common variety of malfunction that yield to the simple techniques of sight training, or are so deep-seated that they require psychotherapy—you *can* improve your vision, and probably rid yourself of your glasses forever. Good luck.

APPENDIX

WHAT THE TITLES MEAN

Anyone who has ever bought eye glasses or has been treated for eye problems is likely to have had difficulty distinguishing among opticians, optometrists, oculists, and ophthalmologists.

An **optician** is a skilled technician who grinds and sells optical lenses according to prescription, as a pharmacist prepares and sells medication according to prescription.

An **optometrist** is a professional man, although not a medical doctor, who measures the extent and determines the character of eye defects, and prescribes corrective lenses. He does not treat pathological conditions.

An **oculist** is a medical doctor who treats the eyes. He does not necessarily have special training in eye care beyond that given all medical students.

An **ophthalmologist** is a medical doctor who has had several years of special training in treating the eyes and who has passed an examination given by a board of eye specialists.

YOUR CHILDREN'S EYES

Readers ask whether children can use the sight training approach presented in this book. My answer is an emphatic yes. One of the most wonderful things about childhood is that change is still relatively easy, even when the child's vision problems seem fairly severe.

When C. was brought to me, she was eight and a half years old. She came with an ophthamologist's diagnosis of cone and color disfunction, photophobia and congenital nystagmus (in which the eyes look as if they are constantly jumping). She was also said to be hyperkinetic, that is, extremely restless. Of course this had produced problems in school since she had trouble just sitting still, let alone learning to read.

In our very first session, I taught her how to gain some control over her restlessness by doing the Long Swing. I did it with her, resting my hands on her shoulders and guiding the swing slowly and continuously from side to side for a count of twenty. She said she felt quiet inside for the first time that she could remember. She became so relaxed, in fact, that she could barely stay awake to get home!

At home she practiced Swinging, Palming and Sunning. She also learned fusion techniques from me, using first a twelve-inch ruler and working up to a yardstick. By the fourth session she was ready for the imaginary dot technique, very important for controlling nystagmus. I accompanied all the visual exercises with much gentle touching of her shoulders to promote relaxation and a sense of being cared for.

At the end of our work together, she had lost her extreme restlessness and was able to focus both her eyes and her attention on a book.

In all of my work with children, I have found that releasing them from the pressure they feel to achieve— teaching them to relax, comforting them and accepting them as they are—leads to a happier child who is able to achieve more with much less struggle and pain. This growth is beautiful to see.

Infants begin to focus their eyes about six weeks after birth, but do not achieve sharp focus until they are 18 months old. To help a child develop focus, and easy eye movements, hang over its crib a brightly colored mobile that swings freely and gently in the slightest motion of the air. Its slow gyrations will discourage staring and encourage full use of the eye muscles.

If the eyes manifest a cast at nine months, pass a lighted flashlight in front of them slowly for a minute at a time three times a day. Keep moving the light in the direction in which you want the eye with the cast to look. Moving from the easy to the difficult, gradually increase this moving rhythm to three minutes at a time three times a day. The child will automatically shut his or her eyes, but the light will do its work anyway, penetrating the delicate eyelids.

After using the flashlight, seat yourself in a rocking chair with the baby on your lap, and rock gently in front of a lighted pole lamp about three feet away. Start with a 40-watt bulb and work up gradually to a 150-watt bulb. Infants love the procedure, which helps not only to correct casts but to calm overactive children.

If the cast persists to the age of two, or appears at that time, induce the child to do the Crawl—something it probably has only recently abandoned for walking. Get down on the floor yourself and show the child how: lie flat on your belly and haul yourself forward with one arm and then the other, legs and hips following arms. Make a game of it and get the child to imitate you. This unlikely procedure stimulates parts of the brain that may not be functioning adequately and that are responsible for the cast.

Where a cast is found at about age four, roll a ball on the floor repeatedly in the direction you want the eye with the cast to shift. Again, make a game of it, passing the ball back and forth between you and the child, and encouraging the child to keep both eyes on it wherever it goes.

Several other techniques also may be used with four-year-olds. Place a patch over the child's good eye and allow him to watch television for no more than 15 minutes with the less effective eye.

At other times, wave a handkerchief or a Christmas

tree ornament or a ball in front of the child in the direction in which the eye lacks mobility, and tell the child: "Talk to your eye. Tell it to follow the handkerchief" (or the ball). Do this for a few minutes several times a day if possible.

In a variation of the procedure, hold up and center a pencil in front of the child and ask him to look beyond it toward a ball while he talks to his unwilling eye. Convince him that it is an engaging trick: "See the two pencils when you look at the ball?"

Children who have had normal eyes in their early years frequently become myopic—nearsighted—at age six, when they go to school. Do not hasten to fit them with eyeglasses. If they cannot read the blackboard at school, let them move closer to it, and give the child more assurance and support. Myopia at that stage in life is merely the result of a muscular spasm and is not yet entrenched: it will pass, or it may be corrected by the techniques recommended elsewhere in this book for myopia. When myopia appears during adolescence, let the parent of the same sex as the child guide the child through sexual trauma.

I know two brothers who became myopic at age six and whose parents immediately bought glasses for them. One brother, an acquiescent child, wore his glasses and, now in his fifties, still does. He is still myopic. The other, more self-assertive, refused to wear glasses and has, since his brief early myopia, enjoyed excellent sight without glasses.

Hyperopia—farsightedness—in children is related to

difficulties in learning and reading. Work patiently at home with the child to help him or her master problems in school. Give the training in perception and memory described in Chapter 6. Teach your child to glide the eyes over a printed page without trying to read.

But bear in mind that many eye defects in children have a psychological basis. Of course, the best therapy of all is to live and grow in such a way that one never needs therapy. Parents can help children avoid visual malfunctions that may need correction later on by encouraging in their children both self-expression and acceptance of a measure of discipline. Induce your children to speak their minds rather than to conceal their rages and resentments and frustrations.

Your children depend on you in so many ways: for their physical needs, for their inner sense of well being. These are natural, healthy dependencies. You have a unique opportunity to open their eyes and all of their senses to the world around them. Teach them to appreciate their senses and use them consciously. Encourage them to feel the different textures in the things they touch, for example. Often touch your children with warmth, embrace them, teach them to express affection without embarrassment.

Perhaps you feel embarrassed to touch or look closely at others. As you become more aware of your own feelings, you may find that these simple ideas are rather difficult to act on. At some point in your own childhood, you got the message that physical and even visual contact with others was wrong. Now is the time, for your children's sake, to experiment with another point of view, in spite of your embarrassment. You are very likely to discover a much more exciting world out there than you were allowed to see as a child. This is the precious gift you can give to your own children: they will not have to be crippled as you may have been.

ACKNOWLEDGMENTS

I want to express appreciation to:

My dear husband, Arnold Berrett, physician and neuroradiologist. Out of an interest and regard for the care of his patients, he has x-rayed eyes and learned to understand the functioning of vision. He has influenced my progress in this work, and improved his own sight as well.

My son, Alan Rosanes, who as a little boy secretly hid himself under the couch to "watch mother work." He is still excited about this work, and has influenced many to learn about it. Frequently, when I thought of giving up, the thought of how disappointed he would be made me continue.

My great mentor, friend, and client, the father of Gestalt Therapy, Dr. Frederick S. (Fritz) Perls, who taught me so much about one's desire to see or not to see oneself and others. He showed me how to apply Gestalt

Therapy. He was my model patient, one who improved his own vision most dramatically.

Dr. T. Earle Moore, who from 1954 to 1957 employed me to conduct group classes in improving sight at his clinic in Miami, Florida.

Dr. Zygmont A. Piotrowski, the Rorschach scientist, and author of *Perceptanalysis,* who encouraged me to note differences in the way myopes and hyperopes handle anxiety.

My many clients who improved their vision under my tutelage, as well as to those who failed to improve and thus made me question, and so advanced my studies in my quest for answers.

Marilyn B. Rosanes-Berrett